Occupational Therapy
for Children with Special Needs

Occupational Therapy for Children with Special Needs

Occupational therapy for children with problems in learning, co-ordination, language and behaviour

Elaine B. Wilson

with Helen Edwards, Joanna Nicklin and Jenny Bennett
in association with Catherine McDerment

W

Whurr Publishers

©1998 Whurr Publishers Ltd
First published 1998 by
Whurr Publishers Ltd
19b Compton Terrace, London N1 2UN, England

British Library Cataloguing-in-Publication Data
A catalogue record for this book is available from the
British Library

ISBN 1 86156 061 3

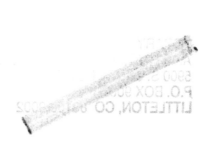

Printed and bound in Malta by Interprint Ltd.

Contents

The authors   xi
Acknowledgements   xv
Preface   xvii
Foreword   xix

Chapter 1 Background to sensory integration – *Elaine B. Wilson*   1
Definitions
Which children might benefit from treatment?
What are the potential benefits of treatment?
Conclusion
References

Chapter 2 Assessment procedures – *Helen Edwards*   6
Defining the problem
Assessment procedures
Ethical considerations
Assessment rationale
Selecting assessment tools
Referral and identification
Pre-assessment organisation
Background history
Test environment
Reporting
Screening tests
Non-standardised tests
Standardised tests
Tests of visual perception
Tests of self-esteem
Tests of handwriting ability
Conclusion
References and recommended reading

Chapter 3 The treatment session – *Elaine B. Wilson*   32
How many children can you treat at once?
Blocks of treatment
Regression effects
Precautions
Positive reinforcers
Difficulties that may arise in any treatment session
Management of behaviour in the treatment session
Parents' role in therapy
Treatment session
Lack of progress
Managing specific deficits
Treating children with other disabilities
Conclusion
References and recommended reading

Chapter 4 Behaviour management in young children: 79
a therapist's guide for parents –*Joanna Nicklin*
Meeting with parents
Family dynamics
Tools of management

Chapter 5 Food and chemical sensitivities –*Jenny Bennett*   89
My story
Sensitivity symptoms
Food
Chemicals
Bathing and cleaning
Altering the home
A day in the life of a child who is food- and chemical-sensitive
Conclusion
References and recommended reading

Appendix 1.1   Instruments for the assessment of children   100
Appendix 1.2   Checklist: the child with learning and co-ordination   102
                   problems
Appendix 1.3   Occupational Therapy Parent Questionnaire   105
Appendix 1.4   Sample letter to accompany School Questionnaire   113
                   Occupational Therapy School Questionnaire   114
Appendix 1.5   Screening guide for Irlen Syndrome   117
Appendix 1.6   Occupational Therapy Referral Form   119
Appendix 1.7   Occupational Therapy Report   120
Appendix 1.8   Sample letter   125
Appendix 1.9   NEED perceptual – Motor Checklist   126

Appendix 1.10 Part 1: Clinical Observations Test   127
                 Part 2: Comments and directions for Clinical   130
                 Observations Test

Appendix 1.11 NEED Centre Observation of Writing   135

Appendix 2 Activities for sensory integrative   137
treatment procedures
Vestibular-proprioceptive
Tactile
Tone
Bilateral activities
Prone extension
Supine flexion
Balance and trunk rotation
Crossing the midline
Unilateral activities
Protective extension
Eye tracking
Eye–hand co-ordination
Motor planning
Visual space perception
Hyperactivity

Appendix 3 Home programme   144
Equipment
Home programme for you to use with your child
Activities

Appendix 4 Equipment   159
Treatment room
Sources of equipment
Assessment tests

Appendix 5 Food challenge handout   187
Foods allowed
Foods to be removed for 14 days
Reintroduction
Antidote
Suggested menu plan
Recommended reading

Glossary   197
Index   201

If we can't behave, we have no friends.
If we are clumsy, we are teased and can't play.
If we can't be understood, we don't socialise.
If we can't understand, we don't learn.
If we can't learn, we don't reach our potential.
If we can't _____ we don't fit in.

To the memory of my mentor and friend, Dr A. Jean Ayres, from whom I gained most of my original knowledge.

The Authors

Elaine Wilson

Elaine Wilson graduated from the Sydney School of Occupational Therapy in 1956 and obtained her Bachelor of Applied Science (Occupational Therapy) from Western Australian Institute of Technology in 1977. In 1978 she was made a faculty member of Sensory Integration International, USA and is now a consultant faculty member of Sensory Integration International in Australia.

Elaine was awarded a six-month Churchill Fellowship in 1973, which enabled her to study sensory integration theory and practice with Dr A. Jean Ayres, both at the University of Southern California and at Dr Ayres' treatment clinic. Since that time, she has attended a number of postgraduate courses in sensory integration in USA. As a result of her extensive experience, she has conducted numerous workshops in every state in Australia, in New Zealand and Hong Kong, and has taught this work at the schools of Occupational Therapy in Perth and Sydney.

Elaine has worked as a clinician treating children of all ages with learning and/or co-ordination problems since 1973, and exclusively since 1981. She has gained a wealth of experience from these last 25 years of practice, and this has encouraged her to disseminate the information contained in this book. In Australia, she is regarded as one of the most experienced occupational therapists in this field of sensory integration.

Helen Edwards

Helen Edwards completed her first degree in Occupational Therapy at the University of Queensland in 1972. Since that time, she has worked in Queensland, Tasmania and New South Wales. Helen's postgraduate study at the University of New England led to the completion of a Masters of Education degree and a Graduate Diploma of Adult Education.

She has always been interested in paediatrics, but it has been her specialist interest area since 1977. In 1976 she was introduced to the concepts of sensory integration by Elaine Wilson. Helen's knowledge in the area has been developing since that time through attending training courses, working directly with children, supervising and teaching students and research. She is a member of the Australian faculty of Sensory Integration International.

Helen has an outstanding ability to combine extremely effective clinical skills with a strong academic background.

Joanna Nicklin

Joanna Nicklin graduated from the Sydney School of Occupational Therapy in 1955. She worked in Brisbane and Sydney until her marriage in 1958, when she worked in Addenbrooke's Hospital, Cambridge, UK until the birth of the first of her six children. She returned to work in 1974, working with pre-school deaf children for 18 years, frequently using sensory integrative treatment procedures.

She has also had a private practice in her home, working with parents and their children with developmental delays and behavioural problems, and with pre-school and school-aged children with learning disabilities. She retired in 1992.

Joanna has exceptional skills for managing children with behavioural problems and the personal and professional experience to advise parents on a very practical level. She plans to write a book for parents.

Jenny Bennett

Jenny Bennett was diagnosed as food and chemical intolerant in 1981. After 30 years of unexplained illness, the new awareness set Jenny on a trail to investigate practical alternatives to the offending food and household chemicals. Many therapists now find that learning, co-ordination, speech and language or behaviour-related problems lessen, or even disappear, after food and/or chemical intolerances have been eliminated.

Jenny travelled to America three years after her intolerances had been diagnosed for further research. Later, in Sydney and Melbourne, over the next few years, she kept in contact with doctors, continued phone assistance, counselled others and attended conferences. In 1987 she wrote *The Allergy Survival Kit*, a book that drew together essential technical, scientific, medical and practical information. In 1988 Jenny visited environmental units in England and met with doctors who were treating food- and chemical-intolerant patients.

On her arrival back in Australia, Jenny was approached by doctors to act as Education Officer at a Special Environmental Allergy clinic in a private Sydney hospital. As a speaker, she covers all age groups, including infant and early childhood, teaching simple, practical, inexpensive and successful methods of survival for affected people and families.

Jenny also has a special interest in children and, as a mother of three, has developed easy methods to prepare food for families with food intolerances. Her ideas led to the writing of a unique book, *The Allergy Tucker Box,* which features meal preparation and integrates special diets with family meals.

Since 1983 she has coupled extensive research both in Australia and overseas with personal and professional experience as an environmental consultant.

Acknowledgements

I wrote this book, with the help of others, as an offering of appreciation to the profession that has given me a most enriched and rewarding life as an occupational therapist.

I wish to thank my co-authors, Helen Edwards, Joanna Nicklin and Jenny Bennett, for their valuable contributions – the time they gave in writing their chapters and the help they gave me with my own writing. I value our personal friendship and the mutual respect that we have for our individual specialties. Each author's work is based on her own experience. I am most appreciative of Catherine McDerment's considerable contribution. Without her help and advice, the book would probably not have been published in Britain. I am grateful to her for allowing us to use her list of Assessment Tests in Appendix 4.

Special thanks go to my editor, Dr Gregory Heard. He was a pleasure to work with and inspired me to keep going when I felt totally daunted by this enormous undertaking. I am most grateful to Richard Litchfield for his excellent desk top publishing skills; to Terry Litchfield for his overall support and assistance in project management; to Greg Gibson for the perfection in his artwork and the detailed cutting of my photographs; to Wayne Roberts for his patient hours of photography; to the children, Megan, Jessica and Philip, who were the subjects in the photographs; and to Margaret Griffiths for proofreading the manuscript originally. Without exception, all of these people appeared to enjoy their involvement; their support meant a great deal to me and has been a major inspiration.

I would also like to thank my many professional colleagues and close friends, especially Chris Chapparo, Jill Hummell and Louise French, for taking the time to read, edit and provide constructive comments on the manuscript. Their input was invaluable.

Very special thanks go to 'my children' and their parents. Were it not for them, this book would never have been possible. They have taught me so much.

Elaine B. Wilson

Preface

This book has been written to help occupational therapists and others working with children who have problems with learning, co-ordination, speech and language, and behaviour. Our aim is to provide practical procedures for working with these children and their families.

The book presents a model of a recognised approach from which therapists and others can develop specific techniques within a clinical setting, modifying the programme to meet the needs of the individual child.

Once, when lecturing to a group of postgraduate occupational therapists in Hong Kong, I was asked to give recipes for treatment. Knowing it was impossible, I said, 'Does anyone here play bridge?' Half the group did, so I replied that treating children is like playing bridge. No two hands are alike, and no two children have exactly the same problems – there are no recipes. However, treatment, like bridge, can be based on principles and past experience.

Occupational therapy using sensory integrative treatment procedures is widespread and well accepted throughout many countries in the world. In the past 20 years, we have treated hundreds of children in this way:

> Clinical research and literature have supported occupational therapy intervention in using neurosphysiological and multisensory developmental principles for the facilitation of sensory integration in such areas as learning disabilities . . . Clinical research had led to the development of evaluation and treatment methodologies that continue to be examined and modified in response to ongoing research. (American Occupational Therapy Association, 1982, p. 831.)

Whilst this book is based on our own experiences and individual skills, we acknowledge that there are many other helpful approaches. We chose not to include a neurophysiological rationale for treatment because the field of brain function and sensory perception is altering rapidly and neurophysiological research is ever-changing. We believe that treatment principles and practice have not altered substantially. Our longitudinal clinical experience and observations, and the present literature (Gorga, 1989; Haradon *et al.*, 1994; Tickle-Degman and Coster, 1995), suggest that benefit can be gained from using sensory integration as part of the overall treatment plan. Tickle-Degman and Coster (1995) have reported that significant functional outcomes may be attributed to sensory integrative therapy, including the ability to initiate, participate in and manage challenging activities (p. 124).

We strongly believe that this treatment complements other aspects of programmes for children, such as remedial teaching and speech therapy. Children who have specific learning difficulties can benefit significantly from this extra assistance.

In this book, we cover the basic deficits commonly seen; the expected outcomes from and benefits of a sensory integrative approach; screening tools and many assessments, both non-standardised and standardised; treatment details, using sensory integrative procedures; the management of behaviour seen in young children (aberrant behaviour being observed in many children who have other problems and therefore being a common reason for initial referral); and practical information on food and chemical sensitivities, which are often a major contributory factor for these patterns of behaviour.

The appendices include referral forms, questionnaires, assessments and report forms; suggestions for treatment activities; the home treatment programmes; equipment used in treatment; a food challenge handout; and a glossary. *Any information in the appendices may be reproduced with acknowledgement.*

The occupational therapist, who is often the lynchpin in a multidisciplinary team, is responsible for endeavouring to see that the overall needs of the children and families are met. We encourage readers to use this book as a basis for ongoing learning. We urge them to seek further knowledge and pursue relevant training to broaden their skills in order to ensure that optimum quality care is provided for these children and their families.

Elaine B. Wilson
Binnaway, NSW
June 1998

References

American Occupational Therapy Association (1982) Occupational therapy for sensory integrative dysfunction. *American Journal of Occupational Therapy* 36(12): 831–4.

Gorga D (1989) Occupational therapy treatment practices with infants in early intervention. *American Journal of Occupational Therapy* 43: 731–6.

Haradon G, Bascom B, Dragomir C, Scripcaru V (1994) Sensory functions of institutionalised Romanian infants: a pilot study. *Occupational Therapy International* 1 (4): 250–60.

Tickle-Degman L, Coster W (1995) Therapeutic interaction and the management of challenge during the beginning minutes of sensory integration treatment. *Occupational Therapy Journal of Research* 15(2): 122–41.

Foreword

We live in an era in which our profession faces a shortage of experienced occupational therapists to serve as role models, supervisors and mentors for newer therapists. This is particularly the case in the practice area of occupational therapy for children with learning, co-ordination, language and behaviour problems. Over the years, therapists have turned to seminal texts such as Jean Ayres' *Sensory Integration and Learning Disorders* (1972), *Sensory Integration and the Child* (1980) and, more recently the work by Fisher, Murray and Bundy, *Sensory Integration: Theory and Practice* (1991), for theoretical and treatment guidance. This book offers therapists a different perspective on the management of children with learning, co-ordination and behaviour problems. It is not a 'text' in a theoretical sense but rather a treatment guide. It contains a compilation of stories, ideas, perspectives and information that is built on the mastery, skills and experience of four therapists who are considered 'experts' in the area.

The emphasis of this book is on practical aspects of intervention. Chapters 1 and 3 outline intervention from a sensory integrative perspective as interpreted by Elaine B. Wilson. In Chapter 2, Helen Edwards reviews existing forms of assessments for children with learning and co-ordination problems, and touches on the ethical and practical aspects of assessment, reviewing the results with parents and children and formal reporting. In Chapter 4, Joanna Nicklin's narrative provides a practical model for guiding parents and therapists in managing difficult behaviours in children with learning and co-ordination problems. In the remaining chapter, Jenny Bennett gives a personal and practical account of how foods and chemicals may contribute to disorders in behaviour.

Research has illustrated that students and clinicians value clinical techniques and their applications. Research also indicates that students and therapists benefit from the wisdom and experience of expert therapists as found in narrations of their own perspectives of the therapy process. From their own life experiences as expert therapists, Wilson, Edwards, Nicklin and Bennett have provided us with a book that is rich in practical ideas for therapy that can be applied to a variety of clinical settings.

Chris Chapparo, PhD DipOT, MA, OTR, FAOTA
Senior Lecturer, School of Occupational Therapy
The University of Sydney, Australia

Chapter 1
Background to Sensory Integration

Elaine B. Wilson

Sensory integration is a treatment approach that has been shown clinically to give children with specific learning difficulties a chance to achieve their full potential.

However, it must be appreciated that these concepts are only hypotheses and thus yet to be proved. Fisher *et al.* (1991) substantiate this and refer to 'hypotheses versus fact'. They suggest the need for empirical research to provide a theoretical basis for sensory integration and appreciate that it is being revised and modified as new knowledge emerges (p. 6).

We have chosen not to include a neurophysiological rationale for treatment (see Preface) in recognition of the changing nature of the knowledge in this area. However, we strongly recommend that readers explore these theoretical aspects through a text that deals fully with current thinking, for example, Fisher *et al.* (1991).

In this chapter, we will look at how sensory integration fits into the jigsaw of the child's nervous system. The following definitions may help the reader to understand these concepts.

Definitions

Sensory input

Sensory input – of movement–pressure, touch, vision, hearing, taste and smell – goes to the brainstem from our sensory organs, mostly via the cranial nerves. All sensory input needs to be registered at the brainstem level.

Sensory registration

Sensory registration which is basic to sensory integration, occurs when the sensory input has been registered in the nervous system.

Sensory integration

Sensory integration, which is basic to sensory perception, is the ability to organise (or integrate) sensory information (or input) at the brainstem level. We perceive and learn through our senses, and sensory input precedes a motor output. There are five times as many sensory fibres as there are motor fibres. Sensory integration affects the efficiency of higher centre function after the sensory information has been processed. There is more efficient brain output when both hemispheres work together.

The developing human brain must have optimum brainstem sensory integration for higher levels to function efficiently. The process is illustrated below.

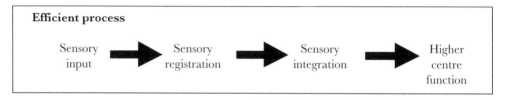

Sensory integrative dysfunction

Sensory integrative dysfunction occurs when sensory integration is inefficiently processed at the brainstem level, affecting the overall higher centre function and subsequent motor output. A dysfunction in one area of the brain will affect the performance in other areas.

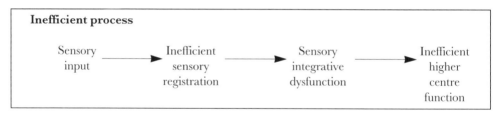

Sensory integrative treatment procedures

Sensory integrative treatment procedures assist in controlling sensory input integrated at the brainstem level, resulting in an improved motor output. Treatment also facilitates the functioning of other areas of the brain involved in learning, co-ordination, speech, expressive and receptive language, and behaviour.

It should be noted that this is a simple model. More complicated combinations are possible, for example where the sensory input is efficient but other stages are not.

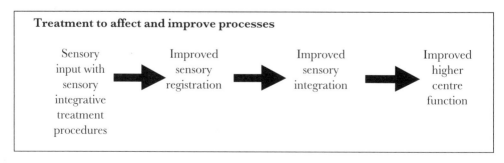

Disinhibition

Disinhibition can manifest itself as overactivity, abnormal irritability, tactile defensiveness, distractibility, poor concentration and memory, fussiness, bedwetting and intolerance to noise, light, smell and movement. Any of these behaviours, particularly overactivity, are common reasons for parents to seek help for their children. Disinhibition can accompany any of the deficits discussed. The author's clinical experience has indicated that disinhibition is closely associated with attention deficit disorder.

Attention deficit disorder

Children with attention deficit disorders (ADD) are quite frequently referred to occupational therapists for assessment of their motor performance. Doyle *et al.*'s (1995) research suggested a need for therapists to be aware that inattention and impulsiveness may be causal factors in apparent motor difficulties. Where motor difficulties are identified, they recommend that therapists, 'assist children to develop strategies to control behaviour, modify impulsiveness, develop self-control and improve attention and effort to task' (p. 238).

Which children might benefit from treatment?

The children who will be discussed are those of normal intelligence, who have a specific learning difficulty, with or without deficits in motor skills, speech, expressive and receptive language, and behaviour, but who have no marked physical disability or 'hard' neurological signs. The deficits that may be encountered in such children are summarised in Table 1.1.

Minimal difficulties revealed in assessment

Sometimes only minimal difficulties may be seen when using the clinical observations assessment in children of any age, particularly those who are 12 years and over who have been referred for specific learning difficulties and may well benefit from treatment. They may have the necessary muscle strength to perform the tests yet have poor sensory integration. The Bruininks–Oseretsky Test of Motor Proficiency (BOTMP) can be used up to 14:6 years and, if one uses one's knowledge of neurological signs, these signs are often evident in the child's performance in the BOTMP test. However, the clinical observations assessment is not sensitive for teenagers, in particular. Therefore it can be difficult for therapists to note any specific deficits as a basis for treatment. Reassure teenagers that it is 'OK' to be doing these tests or to be attending the treatment sessions in future. Make the tests (and later treatment) enjoyable, challenging and age-appropriate.

Table 1.1: Deficits that may respond to sensory integrative treatment procedures

Any inefficient tactile, vestibular-proprioceptive processing, as well as:

Poor balance
Poor bilateral motor co-ordination
Reluctance to cross an imaginary midline of the body
Disinhibition – overactivity, abnormal irritability, distractibility, poor concentration and memory, fussiness, bedwetting, intolerance to light/smell/noise/movement
Poor fine motor co-ordination
Poor fine visual space perception
Gravitational insecurity
Poor gross motor co-ordination
Poor gross motor planning
Poor gross visual space perception
Low muscle tone
Non-conforming behaviour patterns – low in self-esteem and confidence, manipulative and generally difficult to manage at school or at home
Poor prone extension posture
Poor reciprocal motor co-ordination
Unclear speech, difficulty with expressive language, difficulty with receptive language
Poor supine flexion posture
Tactile defensiveness

Your assessment of a child may reveal the presence of single or multiple deficits that cause the child minor or major problems.

What are the potential benefits of treatment?

The objectives of treatment are to provide activities that stimulate the systems responsible for the dysfunctions and to improve the deficits that were identified during the initial assessment. Improvements may occur in any of the following areas (listed alphabetically):

- academic performance
- behaviour, including tactile defensiveness
- concentration
- co-operation with siblings and parents
- gross and/or fine motor co-ordination and motor planning
- independence in self-care skills
- self-confidence
- self-esteem
- speech and language (both expressive and receptive).

Conclusion

Not all children respond to therapy, but research findings and clinical experience suggest that children who have tactile, vestibular-proprioceptive processing problems, with a hyporeactive postrotary nystagmus, usually respond favourably to sensory integrative treatment procedures. Some children respond only after the block of treatment sessions ends. Retesting during a block and/or at the end of a block often reveals improvements in scores.

If your assessment of a child reveals no strongly specific deficits but that child is referred for any of the following reasons – learning disabilities, problems with co-ordination, speech, expressive or receptive language, or behaviour – still treat the child but monitor carefully what is happening. Some children will improve in other areas – behaviour, concentration, self-confidence, self-esteem and quality of life – but not academically. The improvements may start a positive cycle of success → reinforcement → continue to try harder → success → reinforcement.

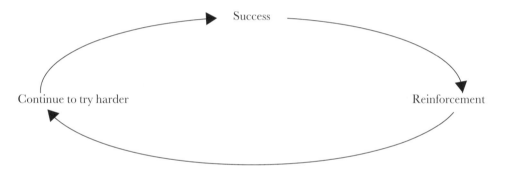

References

Doyle S, Wallen M, Whitmont S (1995) Motor skills in Australian children with attention deficit hyperactivity disorder. *Occupational Therapy International* 2: 229–240.
Fisher A G, Murray EA, Bundy AC (1991) *Sensory Integration: Theory and Practice*. Philadelphia: Davis.

Chapter 2
Assessment Procedures

Helen Edwards

Defining the problem

The problem faced by children with subtle co-ordination difficulties is summed up well by Wilson *et al.* (1992b) as follows:

> The problem is often associated with far more devastating difficulties in social situations, loss of self-confidence and motivation, communication impairment, difficulties in activities of daily living and academic problems. (p. 775)

Although the presenting dysfunction often relates to motor or co-ordination difficulties, the impact is often far more widespread on the child. If the delay in skills is mild, many of these children may catch up with their peers over time, without treatment. However, those with moderate or severe deficits may continue to have problems throughout schooling (Ehrhardt *et al.*, 1987) and possibly for the whole of their life (Parham, 1990).

Results of a 10-year follow-up study by Losse *et al.* (1991) indicated that current screening and assessment tools were of variable merit. They recommended examining the validity, objectivity, reliability and standardisation of each test.

Assessment procedures

> Tests yield numbers, and numbers can do things that words or ideas cannot. In occupational therapy, measurement is central to differential diagnosis, gain or loss assessment, establishing client status, predicting response to therapy, building and testing theory, and conveying information across fields. It is difficult to accomplish any of these goals without some form of measurement. (Ayres, 1989, p. xi.)

The description of measurement by Ayres, defined the approach to be followed in this chapter. The process also involves gathering information about the child; this information is combined into a meaningful whole through the interpretation and reporting process.

This chapter will examine the following aspects of the assessment process: ethical considerations, assessment rationale, selecting assessment tools, referral and identification, pre-assessment organisation, background history, test environment, reporting, screening tests, non-standardised tests, standardised tests, tests of visual perception, tests of self-esteem and tests of handwriting ability.

The occupational therapist's role is to identify and diagnose children with, or at risk of, a developmental or specific learning difficulty related to a motor deficit. The purpose of assessment is to establish whether the child needs direct or indirect services and/or referral to other professional services. Assessment of information processing and perceptual motor abilities provides vital parameters in understanding and planning remedial programmes for people with learning disabilities (Kirk and Gallagher, 1983; Smith, 1983; Lerner, 1985; Cratty, 1994). Typically, the focus of assessment is on perceptual, motor, behavioural and environmental factors. It examines the daily strengths and needs of the children at home, work and play (American Occupational Therapy Association, 1991). Researchers have also called for the development of tools to measure the social–psychological compensations required to perform physically (Cratty, 1994).

Ethical considerations

Assessment tools, plus your knowledge, training and experience, are used to decide on treatment (Farley *et al.*, 1991). Consider the validity and reliability of the instrument when you select and interpret test results (Ernarsson-Backes and Stewart, 1992). Good validity indicates that the scores of a test can be interpreted for the intended purposes. Reliability takes two main forms: interrater and test–retest.

Interrater reliability shows the degree to which different examiners could expect to get similar scores using the test on the same child. Test–retest reliability examines whether or not a child's test scores would be constant over time if retested at a later date.

If you use unreliable tests without established validity, you risk making unethical decisions (Campbell, 1981); the use of such instruments can lead to inaccurate determinations of such things as 'Which child requires treatment?', 'For how long?', and 'What type?' (Lambert, 1988). Justification of treatment and documentation of outcomes are virtually impossible without the appropriate assessment tools (Farley *et al.*, 1991).

Document your evaluations of a child and quantify them wherever possible, so that you have a reference point. Failure to document is not only unethical, but also denies the child's and parents' rights to written information. Such denials are unacceptable and negate service accountability (Edwards *et al.*, 1990).

Assessment rationale

Most occupational therapists adopt a set of assessment procedures to make a differential diagnosis. Ideally, the therapist who will treat the child should conduct the initial assessment, but this is not always possible. Currently there is a wide range of procedures available to therapists. It is unlikely, however, that any one measure will provide all the answers and/or the most appropriate data for interpretation (Foster, 1996).

Explore all avenues, make assessments the foundation for treatment procedures and use strategies that help the children and their families. Many need a great deal of support. They have frequently had the 'run-around' and you may be the end of the line; be careful that you are not added to that 'run-around' list. Parents at this stage want constructive suggestions to help their child.

Selecting assessment tools

(See list in Appendix 1.1)

In the past, there has been great emphasis on choosing assessment tools on the basis of their psychometric qualities, proven reliability and validity. Today, there is a growing realisation that outcomes of assessment need to be considered. The crucial question then becomes 'Is the test helpful to you as a therapist?' Hayes, *et al.* (1987) suggest that you examine whether treatment outcomes are affected positively by your assessment. They warn against looking at assessment separately from treatment as, if you consider only the technical aspects of assessment, you lose sight of the whole person in context.

Psychometric qualities (validity and reliability) reveal how the tool is structured. The importance of being aware of these qualities is discussed above. However, they do not always give insight into how functional the tool will be. Hayes *et al.* (1987) go so far as to say that there could be times when an assessment tool has little or no demonstrated reliability or validity but proves to be very useful for treatment planning. Many of the early versions of clinical observations could possibly be seen this way.

Look beyond the psychometric qualities of assessments, but remember that the tools with good reliability and validity will probably be the most useful in planning treatment (Hayes *et al.*, 1987).

The ability to consider assessed abilities in the context of occupational performance is surely the hallmark of occupational therapy. According to Fisher (1992a), therapists must consider:

> how we assess our clients – how we place the evaluation results within context and how we interpret the results given that context. (p. 184)

However, no assessment tool can serve all purposes in assessing children with sensory integrative dysfunction. An adequate picture of occupational performance can be obtained only if test results, clinical observations, and family and school information are combined.

When you choose assessment tools, consider the following factors:

- what will the results tell me?
- why do I want the information?

- do I need the information?
- how well correlated are the test results and the functional performance of the child? (Fisher, 1992b)

Some tests are reproduced in Appendix 1 and others are available through local suppliers, such as the British Psychological Corporation and NFER Nelson (see Appendix 4). The remaining tests are published in the papers referenced in the bibliography at the conclusion of this chapter. The table in Appendix 1.1: Instruments for the Assessment of Children indicates the author details and the appropriate age range for each.

Referral and identification

Children thought to have specific learning difficulties are often referred to a team of professionals for assessment. The occupational therapist may conclude that sensory integrative treatment procedures are the most effective approach or may elect to use other treatments. The process involved is illustrated in Figure 2.1.

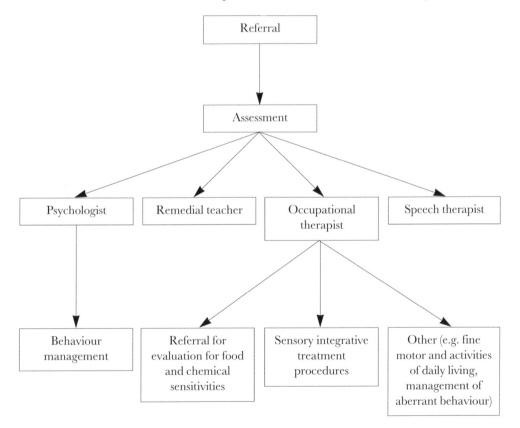

Figure 2.1: Possible pathway after referral

The most common problems and reasons for referral are itemised in a checklist (see Appendix 1.2), which can be completed by parents and/or teachers. Children can have a combination of these problems or have just one or two difficulties that are nonetheless disabling to their overall performance at home, at school and in play.

Ask the family to fill out the Parents' Questionnaire (see Appendix 1.3) as part of the referral process, prior to the day of the assessment. You may ask them to bring in the previous week's food diary in case there is an additional problem of food sensitivity. All this information can help you to interpret the child's history, select appropriate assessments and write the post-assessment report. Send the parents a School Questionnaire with the accompanying letter (see both in Appendix 1.4) for them to take to the teacher if they want the school to be involved. (On rare occasions this is not recommended. If the child or parents are having trouble with the school, they may elect not to notify the school that the child may be treated in occupational therapy. In most centres, it is the parents' choice whether or not they involve the school.) If the referring data indicate a particular difficulty with reading, or spelling and writing, and the child is older than eight years, you may also send a questionnaire for Irlen syndrome (see Appendix 1.5).

Pre-assessment organisation

The procedure prior to assessment involves the acceptance of the referral and the collection of basic details as set out on the Occupational Therapy Referral Form (see Appendix 1.6). If the child cannot be assessed on referral, advise parents of the approximate waiting period. Tell them they will be contacted as soon as the time for assessment is near.

If you have a waiting list for treatment, it may be helpful to assess the child and give the parents a home programme until you have a vacancy. Ideas for the home programme are detailed in Appendix 3.

If the child is overactive or has behaviour problems, it may be appropriate to seek the advice of a psychologist. Alternatively, you may suggest some basic behaviour management strategies (see Chapter 4) and/or a food challenge (see Appendix 5). If the child's difficult behaviour continues, you may investigate chemical sensitivities (see Chapter 5) or refer to a dietician or someone with relevant experience in this field.

Background history

Record the child's history in sufficient detail to indicate the problems as perceived by the parents, the child and the school. An overview from conception onwards will allow you to understand the child in the context of his experiences.

You can collect the history by questionnaire, interview or a combination of these procedures. The child need not be present during the interview, depending on your approach and that of the parents. Make your history questionnaire specific but not so extensive that it threatens parents or provides unnecessary information. Try to have both parents present when you take an oral history. Record each person's perception of the child's problems. When you set goals for treatment and write the post-assessment report, highlight these aspects.

Endeavour to find out what the child thinks are her difficulties – it can surprise you somtimes! Address these accurate (or conceived) problems by talking them through with her. Observe her interaction with others, and, if possible, watch her play. It all helps you to obtain an overall clearer picture of the child.

Recommend vision and hearing screens for the child prior to the assessment or request the reports of any recently completed tests.

Test environment

The environment in which you assess the children can affect their test performance either positively or negatively. For example, if children are doing pencil and paper tasks at desks that are too high, the test scores are unlikely to be a true indication of their abilities. Have a range of chair and table sizes available so that you can adjust the setting to enable the children to sit comfortably (Alston and Taylor, 1984): this means ankles, knees, hips and elbows at 90 degrees.

The examiner's position is also important. When the test requires the examiner to sit beside the child, position the child on your non-dominant side so that you can record scores and comments on test performance out of the child's direct line of vision. There are exceptions; for example, when you observe handwriting, you need to be on the child's non-dominant side or sitting opposite in order to observe adequately such things as grasp, letter shape and formation.

If the test manual indicates that the examiner sits opposite the child, adapt your seating to facilitate eye contact. When working with young children, this may mean that you need to sit on the floor or a very low chair. Otherwise, sit the child on a firm, stable cushion at a regular table and, if necessary, put his feet on a footstool. You must be comfortable so that you can administer the test correctly. Direct eye contact enhances communication and helps to ensure that the child receives your instructions as clearly as possible. It also allows you to pick up additional clinical information about test performance.

Preparation and pre-planning of testing will speed up and enhance the flow of presentation. Have your materials organised and readily accessible. Remove distractors from the test room to enable the child to focus on the task. Set up as much of the test as appropriate without imposing on the setting.

Practise giving a new test to non-dysfunctional children before you use it to diagnose dysfunctional ones. The more difficult the test is to administer, the more children you are advised to practise on. During this 'practice' period, work out a plan for setting up materials (if it is not described in the manual), and always set up the materials in the prescribed way. Create a test environment that will be both comfortable and conducive to optimal performance.

The environment you create around the assessment should be 'fun'. However, you also need to be in a position to control the setting. This can be particularly challenging for a child with poor concentration. A small mat (approximately 610 mm × 460 mm) can be valuable to 'draw' the attention of a distractible child. Direct the child to stand on the mat while you give the test instructions. (Remember to direct rather than ask. If you ask a child to stand on the mat and you are told 'No', respect that choice.) Directing the child does not give the child a choice, and he is more likely to respond as required. Your expectations are obvious to the child, and the limits are clearly defined by the mat. The mat can be particularly useful during gross motor testing of the distractible child.

When you have finished the assessment, ensure that all items of test equipment go back into the test kit in their *correct* places.

Reporting

The written report is a common means of communicating information between professionals and may be your first point of contact; it will leave a lasting impression. Effective report-writing skills are thus worth developing. Vary the style according to your intended audience (Bowman, 1990) (see sample report sheet in Appendix 1.7).

After you complete your assessments, give the parents written, simplified explanations of the rationale behind occupational therapy, stating when you expect the child to commence the programme. Parents appreciate this handout; they can show it to the child's teacher, grandparents and friends. Stress to parents that the child's dysfunction is nobody's fault; some parents feel guilty and blame themselves. Also answer any queries that the parents may have.

After testing, write your detailed report. File one copy and send one copy each to the parents, the school, the local medical officer (if parents give their permission for both of these), and the referring person and any other relevant persons, for example, the psychologist. Reports that you prepare primarily for a school and parents need very little explanation of neurological involvement. In your reports to doctors, include a more extensive description of possible central nervous system dysfunction (Stallings-Sahler, 1990).

Have a chat or send a letter to the child (see the sample letter in Appendix 1.8) with basic explanations of the test results. Write reports to children at their reading and/or comprehension level. Emphasise the positives but do not ignore what the child has found difficult. Use 'kid's talk', such as 'great' or 'not so great' if you wish. Include among your comments an indication of plans for future involvement with the child. However, a letter that only thanks the child for coming and states that you are looking forward to having her for therapy in the near future is still worthwhile. You can also ask children questions at the time of the interview or in a letter, for example 'If I had a magic wand and you could have three wishes, what would you like most?' This can be very informative if the child gives a sincere response.

Remember that you are working in partnership with the whole family, including the child:

> When parents relinquish part of the day, time, care and education of their child to school and teachers, they do not relinquish their parental concerns, or indeed, their parental rights. They are entitled to expect honest, straightforward information, given in a friendly pleasant way. Ignorance about what is really happening at school may often be the cause of adverse comments and criticism from parents. (Northern Territory Department of Education, 1990, p. 4.)

These comments apply equally to the occupational therapy setting, no matter where you are working. If you maintain a high level of trust and honesty with the family, the whole process of assessment, treatment and follow-up will be more rewarding and functional for all involved.

Screening tests

The aim of screening is to highlight the features of a child's functioning that may suggest the need for more thorough investigation. The ideal screening test would select only the students who need referral and do so in a way that is practical for parents, teachers, school counsellors and doctors. A form that can be quickly and easily filled in is more likely to be completed. Therapists based in large community facilities, such as schools, typically use screening tests to establish which children require more detailed assessment (Magalhaes et al., 1989).

The following tests are applicable to children of various ages and functional levels. Several of these tests are quite specific, such as Touch Inventory for Elementary School-aged Children (TIE) for tactile defensiveness and the Motor Development Checklist for Infants Stressed Prenatally with Maternal Cocaine Use. Most of the scales look more generally at the child's abilities. The tests are listed in alphabetical order.

Capital Area Treatment Rating

The Capital Area Treatment Rating (CATR; Farley et al., 1991) was developed to help teachers to identify children who required occupational therapy or physiotherapy to benefit from their education. It is appropriate for persons aged between 3 and 21 years with at least one of the following disabilities: cognitive impairment, neurological impairment, visual impairment, hearing impairment, speech–language impairment, autism, pre-school developmental delay and social and emotional disturbance.

The CATR can be completed in approximately 15 minutes. Farley et al. (1991) claim that it is an effective and efficient way of determining treatment needs; it assists, rather than replaces, the therapist.

Infant/Toddler Screening for Everybaby

The Infant/Toddler Screening for Everybaby (ITSE; Miller, 1993a) was designed to screen the cognitive, language, motor and self-care skills, and behaviour of children from birth to 42 months of age. It is administered by the parent in 20 minutes with the collaboration of a therapist who observes and scores the child.

Infant/Toddler Symptom Checklist

The Infant/Toddler Symptom Checklist (DeGangi et al., 1995) is designed to be used with children from 7 to 30 months of age. Its purpose is to identify young children who are likely to develop sensory integration disorders when they are older. It looks for indicators of attention deficits, emotional, behavioural or learning difficulties. There are six age-specific checklists.

Scotopic Sensitivity/Irlen Syndrome Screen

The Scotopic Sensitivity/Irlen Syndrome Screen (SSIS:Irlen 1991) is used to screen for visual perception difficulties arising because the person does not see the printed page the way proficient readers do. It is a perceptual rather than a visual dysfunction, although regular spectacles are often prescribed to try to deal with the problem. There are many symptoms (see checklist in Appendix 1.5), the most common including rapid eye fatigue; red/watery/aching/stinging eyes from reading; skipping of lines or words; distortions of print; and movement/rapid blurring/doubling/ghosting of print. This can result in significant difficulty with reading, as well as with writing, spelling and maths. People with this syndrome can complain of headaches and/or a marked sensitivity to glare.

An Irlen screen can be carried out by a trained screener, occupational therapist or remedial teacher. It is used for those between the ages of 8 and 80 years and takes approximately 20 minutes to complete. The screener may suggest referral to a trained Irlen consultant, who will perform in-depth assessments for symptoms and, if necessary, prescribe Irlen tinted filters.

Miller Toddler and Infant Evaluation

The Miller Toddler and Infant Evaluation (TIME; Miller, 1993b) is a tool for examining the motor skills of children from birth to 42 months. In the first 18 months of life, the focus is on movement between positions. After 18 months of age, the test looks at motor organisational skills. It aims to evaluate the quality of motor function through observation of transitional movements. Rather than examining individual motor skills, this tool assesses functional performance. It is based on neurodevelopmental and sensory integration theories. The test examines neurological functions, stability, mobility and motor organisation.

A parent interacts and positions the child. The therapist observes the movement between positions and the child's ability to plan motor actions, and scores the performance.

The test requires between 20 and 30 minutes, depending on the age of the child and the experience of the therapist. Pilot editions of the test have demonstrated high levels of test–retest and interrater reliability. Validity studies are planned (Ernarsson-Backes and Stewart, 1992).

Motor Development Checklist for Infants Stressed Prenatally with Maternal Cocaine Use

The Motor Development Checklist for Infants Stressed Prenatally with Maternal Cocaine Use (Cratty, 1994) was designed to identify the motor abilities of infants who had been affected by their mother's use of drugs. It aims to assess abnormal tone, location of tremor and other related motor behaviours and has been reported to have good inter-observer reliability.

Further research is indicated to establish its validity and its use in predicting later developmental problems.

New England Educational Diagnostic Centre Screen

The New England Educational Diagnostic Centre Screen (NEED Screen; Edwards, 1980) uses a quick and simple checklist (see Appendix 1.9) developed by occupational therapists. The checklist, which is based on the work of Gallahue (1976) and on clinical knowledge, is completed by the referring agent. It was designed for use with children attending pre-school through to secondary school. If five or more items on the checklist are identified as being present in the child's functioning, referral is appropriate.

Quick Neurological Screening Test

The Quick Neurological Screening Test (Mooti et al., 1978) groups children into three categories: no deficit, significant neurological signs, and no frank neurological signs but performance below age-appropriate level. Cermak et al. (1986) advised against the use of this tool with children less than 7 years of age owing to reported false-positive identifications in this group.

Screening Test for Evaluating Pre-schoolers

The Screening Test for Evaluating Pre-schoolers (First STEP; Miller, 1992) is a short screen suitable for children aged 2:9 years to 6:2 years. It identifies children who may be developmentally delayed and require more detailed investigation.

The test covers the major developmental areas and can be administered in 15 minutes. The test procedure can be learned from a training video used in conjunction with the manual.

Test of Sensory Functions in Infants

The Test of Sensory Functions in Infants (TSFI; DeGangi and Greenspan, 1989) was designed as a clinical and research tool to screen infants for sensory integrative dysfunction and those at risk of learning disabilities. It is suitable for children aged 4 to 18 months old. Total test scores are reliable and valid, with high inter-observer reliability (Haradon et al., 1994).

Touch Inventory for Elementary School-aged Children

The Touch Inventory for Elementary School-aged Children (TIE; Royeen and Fortune, 1990) detects tactile defensiveness in school-aged children. It takes approximately 10 minutes to complete.

Non-standardised tests

Clinical observations

Many occupational therapists regularly augment the information gained from standardised tests with self-designed clinical observations (Bowman, 1990; Richardson *et al.*, 1992). One study reported that as many as 80% of therapists who assessed children with a learning disability made use of clinical observations (Yack, 1989).

Strong support for such use of clinical observations in sensory integration was given by Ayres (1972a, 1976), who always used non-standardised tools in association with her formal testing to obtain a clearer picture of the whole child. Ayres observed muscle tone, prone extension, supine flexion and balance (Fisher and Murray, 1991).

In 1977 Johnson published a clinical observations schedule containing 19 subtests. The administration and scoring procedures were, however, not standardised, the therapist's experience and judgement having a strong influence on such testing (Lunz and Stahl, 1990).

Dunn's research in 1981 on clinical observations carried out in 5- and 6-year-old children revealed variation in performance in this age group. Wilson (1984) found that children between the ages of six and puberty were able to perform these tests with more accuracy, which gave a clearer clinical picture.

Although there has been significant research in the area of clinical observations, no standardised tool has to date been published:

> As an informal assessment, the clinical observation does not have demonstrated reliability or validity but is being used to make decisions about which children exhibit dysfunction and which children may benefit from intervention. (Wilson *et al.*, 1992b, p. 776.)

The lack of objective criteria for scoring and clear standards for administration continue to be cited as important threats to the reliability of current versions of clinical observations (Wilson *et al.*, 1994; McConnell, 1994).

The Clinical Observations protocol (Wilson, 1984) (see test and directions in Appendix 1.10) was based on Wilson's work with Ayres and her own clinical experience. It examined factors such as the ability to inhibit primitive reflexes and assess co-ordination, ocular pursuits, postural stability and movement abilities. It was designed for use with pre-schoolers and primary and secondary school students. However, Wilson (1984), like Wilson *et al.* (1994), reported that the children who had reached puberty were usually so muscularly 'strong' that they performed the tests well despite their problems, particularly with schoolwork and co-ordination.

It takes time and skilled instruction to learn to use this tool effectively. Over time, therapists tend to become more skilled in its use as the 'trained eye' becomes more perceptive. However, inexperienced assessors tend to be inconsistent, lenient and unreliable in the way they use the instrument. Also, some items rely on the therapist's comments rather than a score, so are difficult to quantify. A training video has been made to aid instruction.

The Clinical Observations Test can be completed in 30 minutes. The original protocol developed by Wilson (1984) contained 23 items, represented by 40 sub-items.

McConnell's (1994) study examined the relationship between these clinical observations and children with developmental co-ordination disorders. He recommended the following:

> For the present, occupational therapists should regard items examining diadochokinesia (sic), thumb-finger touching, prone extension posture, postural background movements and observations of trunk rotation, and postural changes in Schilder's arm extension posture are useful when assessing children with suspected developmental co-ordination disorder. (p. 289)

The results of his study suggest that these subtests are the most likely to provide reliable data.

Clinical Observations of Motor and Postural Skills

The original work of Ayres (1976) and Johnson (1977) provided the starting point for the revision and development of the Clinical Observations of Motor and Postural Skills (COMPS: Wilson *et al.*, 1994). The primary purpose of COMPS was to provide a screening tool for motor deficits. The authors hope that, over time, it will also prove useful in predicting problems and gauging change. They state that COMPS assesses cerebellar function, postural control and motor co-ordination.

Test–retest reliability was reported to be excellent. Acceptable consistency and reliability across time and observers were also found. When experienced observers were used, these results were particularly apparent (Wilson *et al.*, 1994). The authors claimed that, with such high internal consistency, the test measures the single construct of skills underpinning movement and posture. Overall, the authors concluded that the test has adequate reliability and construct validity. This conclusion in relation to reliability has been challenged (McConnell, personal communication, 1993) on the basis that it was established with testers other than those implementing COMPS research.

The original COMPS consisted of seven subtests. A clear rationale for selecting these items and eliminating others is not given (McConnell, personal communication, 1993). Because the Schilder's Arm Extension Test did not discriminate well, it was removed from the battery. However, it should be noted that the authors arrived at this conclusion on the basis of analysing the total subtest scores. Had they looked at the five sections of the test individually, the outcome might have been different.

The remaining items in COMPS are slow motion, finger–nose touching, rapid forearm rotation, prone extension posture, asymmetrical tonic neck reflex and supine flexion posture. Skills in these areas are expected to have matured by eight years of age. The test discriminates least well between children from 6 to 7 years of age. The authors postulated that many of the skills assessed by COMPS are maturing rapidly during this period.

If a child is older than 12, he is usually so muscularly 'strong' that he will do all the tests well despite having problems in specific areas such as learning, co-ordination, speech or behaviour.

COMPS can be completed in 20 minutes. It is easy to administer and is enjoyed by the child. The authors showed that it could identify children with motor deficits (Wilson *et al.*, 1994).

The development of COMPS is a step forward in developing clinical observations. However, it is also clear that further research is still needed.

Pediatric Clinical Tests of Sensory Interaction for Balance

The Pediatric Clinical Tests of Sensory Interaction for Balance (P-CTSIB; Richardson *et al.*, 1992) can be used to identify children with balance deficits. The test aims to provide therapists with details of how a child selects sensory inputs and their effect on postural responses. Six different sensory conditions and two foot positions are used. The test requires two examiners and takes approximately 30 minutes to complete.

A study of pre-school children showed that, whereas the subtest involving the 'feet together' position identified children with balance deficits, the heel–toe position had little diagnostic value (Richardson *et al.*, 1992).

Children under the age of 7:6 years tended not to select sensory input in a systematic way (Forssberg and Nashner, 1982). Rather, they tended to move from a reliance on visual input to one on vestibular input for balance tests. Consequently, their performance on tests of balance varied more significantly than did the performances of children in upper primary school.

Standardised tests

To use a standardised test, occupational therapists must first complete the appropriate training on that instrument; test results generated by untrained therapists may be invalid. Standardised tests are generally complex to administer and, unless they are administered accurately, the information obtained may not be sufficiently sound to give a differential diagnosis.

Nine standardised tests are outlined below. It is not unusual to use several of these tools to assess a child. Some require completion of a certification programme prior to use, whereas others can be learnt from the manual. Most of the tests examine performance across a number of areas; a few, such as the Goodenough–Harris Drawing Test and the Southern California Postrotary Nystagmus Test, are quite specific.

Bruininks–Oseretsky Test of Motor Proficiency

The Bruininks–Oseretsky Test of Motor Proficiency (BOTMP: Bruininks, 1978) is standardised with children aged 4:6 years to 14:6 years. The full test takes approximately 1 hour, and the short form 20 minutes. It is valid for use in a test–retest situation to gauge treatment effectiveness. The eight subtests can yield three estimates of motor skills – gross motor, fine motor and a composite of all tests – but use of the individual subtest scores is recommended (Hattie and Edwards, 1987).

One can amass much additional information by observing closely the child's behaviour during testing, although this is not described in the test manual. For example, associated movements can be seen in some children during thumb–finger touching and when cutting out a circle. Failure to cross the midline can be seen in the visual motor subtest. Children with motor planning problems may score well on the visual motor subtest yet exhibit significant adaptive responses. There is no time limit on this subtest, which allows some children to work out a strategy for success.

This test can clearly provide useful data, as long as the examiner has the skill to observe the child's performance in more detail than is prescribed in the manual. Interpretation of the results of the BOTMP is significantly enhanced by a knowledge of sensory integration theory. Significant correlations have been demonstrated between the BOTMP and the Southern California Sensory Integration Tests (SCSIT). More of the fine motor subtests on the BOTMP correlated with the SCSIT than did the gross motor subtests (Ziviani *et al.*, 1982). The overall correlation seemed to indicate a common practic-postural domain (Ayres and Marr, 1991).

The short form of the test was designed for use as a screening tool. Fine (1979) suggested that it not be used to screen and also indicated that examiners required much expertise in order to use and interpret the scores.

Detroit Test of Learning Aptitude – Primary

The Detroit Test of Learning Aptitude – Primary (DTLA-P; Hammill and Bryant, 1986) is standardised for use with children aged 3 to 9. It aims to assess the child's verbal, non-verbal, conceptual, structural, short-term memory, long-term memory, manual dexterity, oral or pointing responses. Some therapists have used this test instead of the SCSIT or SIPT (see below).

Goodenough–Harris Drawing Test

The Goodenough–Harris Drawing Test (Goodenough and Harris, 1963) can be used with groups or individuals. It was standardised with children aged 3 to 15 years and involves the child drawing a picture of a man, woman and him or herself. The test is scored on the basis of body parts and features shown, plus drawing quality.

Assessment before and after treatment with sensory integrative treatment procedures provides data on the child's awareness of body image. This can be useful in discussions of the child's progress with parents and teachers.

Recent research by Short De-Graff and Holan (1992) has shown that a briefer scoring system would be appropriate, particularly for pre-schoolers. They felt that their system would be a valid screening tool for perceptual–motor performance. These authors highlighted the need for revision of the traditional Goodenough–Harris test. Because society's norms and expectations of women have changed markedly in the 30 years since the test was published, the scoring discriminated against some children.

McCarron Assessment of Neuromuscular Development

The McCarron Assessment of Neuromuscular Development (MAND; McCarron, 1982) is standardised for use with persons aged 3:6 years to young adults. The test has been used with children with 'normal' ability, developmental delay, visual impairment and hyperactive behaviour. Norms are also included for adults with neuropsychological disabilities and visual impairment.

The MAND takes approximately 30 minutes to administer. Subtest items include fine motor, gross motor, persistent control, muscle power, kinesthetic integration and bimanual dexterity. Specialised training is required to give this test.

Miller Assessment for Pre-schoolers

The Miller Assessment for Pre-schoolers (MAP; Miller, 1988b) can be used as a screening or diagnostic tool. For screening, it identifies pre-schoolers (2:9 years to 5:8 years) who need further evaluation. As a diagnostic tool, it assists with the development of a profile of the child's abilities and provides direction in treatment planning. The results can be divided into nine categories for specific therapeutic intervention. The data give a picture of the traditional developmental areas as well as the level of neurological development.

The MAP is designed for use by therapists and educators. Administration carried out on an individual basis takes from 25 to 35 minutes. The duration is influenced by the age and developmental status of the child (Miller, 1988c). The test has strong psychometric qualities, including predictive validity for later learning disabilities (Deloria, 1985; Michael, 1985).

A video is available for self-directed learning of the MAP if the test is to be used for screening. Therapists who intend using it in diagnosis should attend an administration and interpretation workshop. When the test is used as a diagnostic tool, it is often in association with other evaluations to develop a broad picture of a child's development (American Occupational Therapy Association, 1991). Miller (1988c) suggested that tests such as BOTMP, VMI, Goodenough–Harris Drawing Test and Test of Visual Perception be used in conjunction with MAP.

Movement Assessment Battery for Children

The Movement Assessment Battery for Children (Movement ABC; Henderson and Sugden, 1992) is reported to be one of the most commonly used assessment tools to identify children with developmental co-ordination disorders (Howard, 1997).

The battery provides qualitative and quantitative data on the factors leading to movement difficulties. It is standardised for use with children ranging in age from 4 to 12 years. Approximately 20 – 30 minutes administration time is involved.

The Movement ABC is composed of three parts: a classroom screening tool, an assessment battery and guidelines to plan management and remediation programmes. The manual also includes a case study section and contributions from occupational therapists and other professionals, describing how Movement ABC has been used in various settings across the globe.

A study by Shoemaker *et al.* (1994) indicated that the Movement ABC provided a reliable measure of a child's disorder. They also suggested that it allowed them to predict the duration of treatment.

Sensory Integration and Praxis Tests

The Sensory Integration and Praxis Tests (SIPT; Ayres, 1989) were designed to diagnose sensory integrative problems, particularly praxis. They were developed to use with children with mild-to-moderate learning, behavioural or developmental dysfunctions, replacing the SCSIT (Kimball, 1990; Ayres and Marr, 1991). Examiners *must* complete a certification course to be eligible to administer the test. The test is standardised for use with children aged 4 years to 8:11 years. It includes 17 subtests, which take approximately 90 minutes to complete.

The SIPT aims to measure aspects of the sensory and neurological processes that underpin behaviour, learning and language, and praxis (Stallings-Sahler, 1990). It has strong predictive validity for academic achievement. The Motor Accuracy subtest is the best single discriminator of dysfunction. Design Copying is the best measure of visuopractic skills (Ayres, 1989). Overall interrater reliability and test–retest reliability for the tests are high (Ayres and Marr, 1991).

The child's test results are forwarded to Western Psychological Services (WPS) in California for computerised scoring and interpretation. The WPS report contains standardised and percentile scores and a comparison of the child's scores, shown graphically, with six standard clusters. The graphed scores are a valuable aid for discussions with parents and teachers. However, the process of computer analysis has added a major cost and time factor to this test.

The manual reports concurrent validity with the Kaufman Assessment Battery for Children (Kaufman and Kaufman, 1983) plus parts of the Luria–Nebraska Neuropsychological Battery: Children's Revision (Golden *et al.*, 1980), BOTMP and Bender–Gestalt Test for young children (Koppitz, 1975). A study conducted by Chu (1996) in London showed that the SIPT can provide useful diagnostic information. It also produced some limited 'norms' for 5 to 8-year-old British children.

Ayres and Marr (1991) recommend that diagnoses should not be made purely on the basis of SIPT scores. Rather, they have indicated the importance of gathering information on the child's history, functioning at home and school, and data from other tests, including clinical observations. Measures of ocular and postural responses, sensory defensiveness and gravitational insecurity were cited as important subtests of the clinical observations to complete. When all this information is linked into the test scores and sensory integration theory, the whole diagnostic picture of the child should be clear. Only then will the test scores become meaningful (Fisher and Bundy, 1991).

Lai *et al.* (1996) have suggested that there is need for a new test with half as many items in it. They also recommend avoiding the use of a computerised scoring system. They state that the new test 'would be more practical for use in clinical practice and could be adopted more readily for use in other countries' (p. 88).

Southern California Postrotary Nystagmus Test

The Southern California Postrotary Nystagmus Test (SCPNT; Ayres, 1975) is a standardised test designed to measure how well a person's nervous system processes movement of the body (Stallings-Sahler, 1990). Owing to the global influences of the vestibular system, Ayres (1972b, 1976, 1980, 1989) recommended that the SCPNT should never be the sole test used and emphasised that it should be included in the total test procedure.

It was initially designed for use in conjunction with the SCSIT and Clinical Observations. The SCPNT has now been incorporated as a subtest of the SIPT (Wiss and Clark, 1990). It was standardised on a sample of children aged 5 to 9 years.

The reliability and validity of SCPNT are adequate when the test is administered by trained, experienced therapists (Wiss and Clark, 1990).

Southern California Sensory Integration Tests

The Southern California Sensory Integration Tests (SCSIT; Ayres, 1972b) were designed for use with physically and intellectually normal children with specific learning difficulties. The battery aimed to detect and identify the nature of sensory integrative dysfunction. The tests were designed to measure visual, tactile and kinaesthetic perception, and perceptual–motor performance.

They are standardised for use with children aged between 4 years and 8:11 years of age. However, the visual perception subtests were standardised with children aged 4 years to 10:11 years. Testing can be completed in one sitting over a 75–90-minute period. Alternatively, it can be administered over two 45-minute sessions. Examiners must complete a certification course to be eligible to administer the test and interpret the results.

Therapists have been advised to use it only as a diagnostic tool and not to measure outcomes of treatment. Post-testing with the SCSIT has not been shown to measure accurately any change in sensory integrative functioning (Kimball, 1990). It does, however, provide useful information on which to base a treatment programme. Even though the SCSIT was developed many years ago, Howard (1997) reported that it is still commonly used. McDerment (personal communication, 1997) reported, however, that, since the introduction of the SIPT, the SCSIT is not in general use in Great Britain.

Tests of visual perception

There is some question about the reliability of the following tests of visual perception but, as clinical assessment tools, they provide useful additional information. When used together, the results usually are consistent.

Developmental Test of Visual–Motor Integration

The Developmental Test of Visual–Motor Integration (VMI; Beery, 1989) aims to assess the child's ability to perceive visually, and to reproduce manually two-dimensional symbols. It is standardised for children between the ages of 2 and 19 years, and is particularly aimed at pre-school and early primary school children. It can be administered to individuals or groups, taking approximately 15 minutes to complete.

When the VMI is used in combination with other assessments, it can help to predict school achievement and reading problems, particularly among 5 to 8-year-old children (Miller, 1990). Reports of reliability and validity suggest that the VMI is relatively high in comparison with other tests of visual perception (Salvia and Ysseldyke, 1991).

Developmental Test of Visual Perception – 2

The Developmental Test of Visual Perception – 2 (DTVP – 2; Hammill et al., 1993) is used to test the visual perceptual skill of children aged 4 to 10 years. The test can be administered in 35 minutes. It consists of eight subtests that measure spatial relations, position in space, form consistency and figure–ground perception. A study by Moryosef-Ittah and Hinojosa (1996) supports the discriminant validity of this test. Their results also suggest that the test's sensitivity increased as the children got older.

Motor Free Visual Perception Test

The Motor Free Visual Perception Test (MVPT; Colarusso and Hammill, 1972) assesses the child's ability to understand what he or she is seeing in terms of spatial relationships, visual and figure–ground discrimination, visual closure and visual memory. The test is standardised for children between the ages of 5 and 8 years. The advantage of this test is that the child is not disadvantaged by poor fine motor skills. The MVPT is noted for its technical qualities (McLoughlin and Lewis, 1986).

Test of Visual–Perceptual Skills (Non-motor)

The Test of Visual–Perceptual Skills (Non-motor) (TVPS; Gardner, 1988) measures visual discrimination, visual memory, visual spatial relations, visual form constancy, visual sequential memory, visual figure ground and visual closure. It was designed to assess children aged 4 years to 12:11 years.

Tests of self-esteem

These tests are not carried out routinely but may be administered halfway through a block of regular therapy if low self-esteem appears to be hindering progress.

Coopersmith Self Esteem Inventories

The Coopersmith Self Esteem Inventories (Coopersmith, 1981) are made up of three self-concept measures: the School Form, the Adult Form and a teacher's scale. Only the School Form is standardised. The norms given apply to children aged 8 to 15 years. The School Form is a checklist of positive and negative statements that are checked by the child. It takes approximately 10 minutes to complete. The examiner may read the items to a child who has difficulty reading. They can be done with groups or individually.

Piers–Harris Children's Self-concept Scale

The Piers–Harris Children's Self-concept Scale (Piers and Harris, 1984) is a self-report checklist. It is standardised for children aged 9–18 years old. The test can be completed in about 20 minutes. Some schools use it as a screening tool to pick up self-concept difficulties. Some therapists use it as a pre- and post-treatment measure of self-concept, or as an informal assessment and to develop local norms (McLoughlin and Lewis, 1986). A modification of the Piers–Harris Scale has been developed by Cratty (1994) as the Self-opinion Questionnaire. His results show positive correlations between children's performance perception and attitudes to play, as well as feelings about their abilities. Similar relationships were shown between actual performance and feelings, and also to play attitudes.

Tests of handwriting ability

Like motor skills generally, handwriting is displayed in a wide variety of ways, with a range of performance in children of similar ages (Pickard and Alston, 1985). If a child's referral problem includes handwriting, you may wish to investigate it in detail. The results of the SIPT will indicate whether the basis of the dysfunction is a somatosensory processing difficulty leading to motor memory problems, or visual form and space analysis delays.

Successful completion of the first nine tests of the VMI is thought to indicate the child had the skills to learn to print (Beery, 1982). Children who had not mastered these items on the VMI showed similar delays on the fine motor tests of the BOTMP, MAP and MVPT (Oliver, 1990).

A study by Tseng and Murray (1994) showed that poor handwriters do not score as well as good handwriters on most perceptual–motor tests. They recommended therapists assessing children with handwriting problems to examine motor planning ability.

Diagnosis and Remediation of Handwriting Problems

The test for Diagnosis and Remediation of Handwriting Problems (DRHP; Stott *et al.*, 1985) provides a systematic way of analysing handwriting problems. It can be administered to individuals or groups in approximately 20 minutes and is designed for use with school-aged children. Alston and Taylor (1984) found the DRHP to be most useful for children who had been learning to write for at least two years.

The test aims to identify the specific problem and its underlying cause. The manual provides scoring methods, although these are intended for research use only.

Handwriting Checklist

The Handwriting Checklist (Alston and Taylor, 1984) covers three areas: prerequisite skills, letter formation and presentation. The information gathered gives a picture of writing performance. However, no scoring procedures have been given as its purpose is diagnostic. It has been shown to have adequate reliability and validity (Alston and Taylor, 1987). It was designed for use with high school children.

Provision is made on the checklist for treatment objectives. The authors recommend regular collection of writing samples from the child in order to monitor progress. They suggest using these as the basis for discussion about the progress being made over time.

The Handwriting File (Alston and Taylor, 1984) was designed to be used with the Handwriting Checklist. It provides information and guidelines for treatment.

NEED Observation of Writing

The NEED Observation of Writing (NOW; Edwards, 1981), is a checklist (see Appendix 1.11), based on indicators of writing problems (Phillips, 1976) and clinical experience at the New England Educational Diagnostic Centre (NEED). The NOW is appropriate for use with children attending primary and high schools. It provides data on how the child approaches the task of handwriting and where errors occur, allowing the observation and description of the various factors involved in handwriting.

No two persons hold a pen in exactly the same way. However, the optimum position for right-hand writing has the whole hand and wrist on the paper. The thumb and first finger are bent to enable the tips to make contact with the pen at a similar point on the pen to that of the second finger – similar to a three-point chuck grip, at approximately 2 cm from the pen tip. The shaft of the pen should rest on the proximal phalanx of the index finger. The metacarpal line should remain constant in relation to the line as the child writes.

Speed of writing is also evaluated. Efficiency is gauged against the following criteria set as average school grade speeds for New South Wales children:

Grade 2: 30 letters per minute; Grade 3: 35 letters per minute;
Grade 4: 40 letters per minute; Grade 5: 50 letters per minute;
Grade 6: 60 letters per minute; Grade 7: 70 letters per minute.
As speed increases, observe whether structure and rhythm are being maintained.

A study by Ziviani and Elkin (1986) established that, on average, girls wrote significantly faster than boys, a finding that should be considered in interpreting the test results.

Conclusion

This chapter has provided an overview of some of the instruments used by occupational therapists to assess the sensory integrative function of referred children.

Supplementary testing has been a hallmark of much sensory integrative assessment, particularly where therapists have not been trained to use the SIPT. The additional tests have been used to gather data about the child's skills through evaluation of, for example, visual perception, self-esteem and handwriting measures. This information has provided a base for the planning of treatment using sensory integrative procedures.

Research must continue in an effort to develop more effective assessment tools, such as Lai et al.'s (1996) study has suggested. Much of the criticism of sensory integrative treatment procedures stems from our failure to have documented change that can be directly attributed to treatment. A report by Howard (1997) has alerted us to the fact the child is still developing. Therapists must therefore take into account the natural progress the child may have made irrespective of treatment.

Currently the theories of occupational science are emerging and influencing the way many therapists work. In relation to children, studies have provided information on the what, how and why of play and its effects on individuals (Parham, 1996). These data have been a valuable resource for therapists.

Occupational therapists have a responsibility to embark on this assessment phase of a professional relationship only if the resources are available to carry out appropriate follow-up treatment indicated by the evaluation (Miller, 1988c).

Assessment outcomes dictate the goals that are set for treatment. Assessment also enables the monitoring of outcomes. Occupational therapists require a variety of tools and procedures to describe successfully these processes (Hagedorn, 1995).

Use assessments that will give a differential diagnosis. There is no point in carrying out assessments that fail to provide pointers for treatment (Levine, 1993). It is also vital that therapists interpret accurately the test results. Vaugh and Lyon (1994) provided the following caution:

Using test scores that 'work' in practice without some understanding of what they mean, is like using a drug that works without knowing its properties and reactions (p. 325).

References and recommended reading

Alston J, Taylor J (1981) *Handwriting Checklist*. Wisbech: LDA.

Alston J, Taylor J (1984) *Handwriting File: Diagnosis and Remediation of Handwriting Difficulties*. Wisbech: LDA.

Alston J, Taylor J (1987) *Handwriting: Theory, Research and Practice*. London: Croom Helm.

American Occupational Therapy Association (1991) Statement: Occupational Therapy provision for children with learning disabilities and/or mild to moderate perceptual and motor deficits. *American Journal of Occupational Therapy* 45(12): 1069–74.

Ayres AJ (1972a) *Sensory Integration and Learning Disorders*. Los Angeles: Western Psychological Services.

Ayres AJ (1972b) *Southern California Sensory Integration Tests*. Los Angeles: Western Psychological Services.

Ayres AJ (1975) *Southern California Postrotary Nystagmus Test Manual*. Los Angeles: Western Psychological Services.

Ayres AJ (1976) *The Effects of Sensory Integrative Therapy on Learning Disabled Children. The Final Report of a Research Project*. Los Angeles: University of Southern California.

Ayres AJ (1978) Learning disabilities and the vestibular system. *Journal of Learning Disabilities* 11: 18–29.

Ayres AJ (1980) *Southern California Sensory Integration Tests Manual*. Revised 1980. Los Angeles: Western Psychological Services.

Ayres AJ (1989) *Sensory Integration and Praxis Tests*. Los Angeles: Western Psychological Sevices.

Ayres AJ, Marr DB (1991) Sensory integration and praxis tests. In Fisher AG, Murray EA, Bundy AC (Eds) *Sensory Integration: Theory and Practice*. Philadelphia: Davis, pp 203–28.

Beery KE (1982) *Developmental Test of Visual–Motor Integration*. Cleveland: Modern Curriculum Press.

Beery KE (1989) Developmental Test of Visual–Motor Integration. 3rd edn. Cleveland: Modern Curriculum Press.

Bowman OJ (1990) Balancing art and science and private and public knowledge: a matrix for successful practice. *American Journal of Occupational Therapy* 44(7): 583–7.

Bruininks RH (1978) *Bruininks–Oseretsky Test of Motor Proficiency Examiners Manual*.Circle Pines: American Guidance Service.

Burgess MK (1989) Motor control and the role of occupational therapy: past, present and future. *American Journal of Occupational Therapy* 43(5): 345–8.

Campbell SK (1981) Measurement and technical skills – neglected aspects of research education. *Physical Education* 61:523.

Cermak SA, Henderson A (1989) The efficacy of sensory integration procedures: Part I. *Sensory Integration Quarterly* 17(3): 1–5.

Cermak SA, Henderson A (1990) The efficacy of sensory integration procedures: Part II. *Sensory Integration Quarterly* 18(1): 1–5.

Cermak SA, Ward EA, Ward LM (1986) The relationship between articulation disorders and motor coordination in children. *American Journal of Occupation Therapy* 35: 782–7.

Chapparo CJ (1985) AAOT position paper on sensory integration. *Australian Journal of Occupational Therapy* 32(1): 25–6.

Chu S (1996) Evaluating the sensory integration functions of mainstream school children with specific developmental disorders. *British Journal of Occupational Therapy* 59(10): 465–74.

Cohen H (1989) Testing vestibular function: problems with the Southern California Postrotary Nystagmus Test. *American Journal of Occupational Therapy* 43(7) 475–7.

Colarusso RP, Hammill DD (1972) *Motor-free Visual Perception Test*. San Rafael: Academic Therapy.

Coopersmith S (1981) *Coopersmith Self-esteem Inventories*. Palo Alto: Consulting Psychologists Press.

Cratty BJ (1994) *Clumsy Child Syndromes: Descriptions, Evaluation and Remediation*. Harwood: Langhorne.

DeGangi GA, Greenspan SI (1989) *Test of Sensory Functions in Infants*. Los Angeles: Western Psychological Services.

DeGangi GA, Poisson S, Santman AS (1995) *Infant/Toddler Symptom Checklist: A screening tool for parents*. San Antonia Psychological Corporation.

Deloria DJ (1985) Review of Miller assessment for preschoolers. In Mitchell JV (Ed). *The Ninth Mental Measurements Yearbook*. Lincoln: University of Nebraska Press.

Doyle S, Wallen M, Whitmont S (1995) Motor skills in Australian children with attention deficit hyperactivity disorder. *Occupational Therapy International* 2: 229–40.

Dunn W (1981) cited in McConnell DB (1994) Clinical observations and developmental co-ordination disorder: Is there a relationship? *Occupational Therapy International* 1: 278–91.

Dunn W (1986) Developmental and environmental contexts for interpreting clinical observations. *Sensory Integration Special Interest Section Newsletter* 9(2): 4–7.

Edwards HE (1980) *NEED Screen*. Unpublished screening tool developed at the New England Educational Diagnostic Centre.

Edwards HE (1981) *NEED Observation of Writing*. Revised unpublished assessment tool developed at the New England Educational Diagnostic Centre.

Edwards H, Llewellyn G, Nicol P (1990) *New England Early Childhood Services: Going Forward into the Nineties*. Unpublished report completed for the Developmental Disabilities Service, Tamworth.

Ehrhardt P, McKinlay IA, Bradley G (1987) Cited in Wilson B, Pollock N, Kaplan BJ, Law M, Faris P (1992) Reliability and construct validity of the clinical observations of motor and postural skills. *American Journal of Occupational Therapy* 46(9): 775–83.

Ernarsson-Backes LM, Stewart KB (1992) Infant neuro-motor assessments: a review and preview of selected instruments. *American Journal of Occupational Therapy* 46(3): 224–32.

Farley SK, Sarracino T, Howard PM (1991) Development of a treatment rating in school systems: service determination through objective measurement. *American Journal of Occupational Therapy* 45(10): 898–906.

Fine DL (1979) Review of the Bruininks–Oseretsky Test of Motor Proficiency. *Journal of Educational Measurement* 16: 290–2.

Fisher AG (1992a) Functional measures. Part 1: What is function? What should we measure and how should we measure it? *American Journal of Occupational Therapy* 46(2): 183–5.

Fisher AG (1992b) Functional measures. Part 2: Selecting the right test, minimising the limitations. *American Journal of Occupational Therapy* 46(3): 278–81.

Fisher AG, Bundy AC (1991) The interpretation process. In Fisher AG, Murray EA, Bundy AC (Eds). *Sensory Integration: Theory and Practice*. Philadelphia: Davis. pp. 234–50.

Fisher AG, Murray EA (1991) Introduction to sensory integration theory. In Fisher AG, Murray EA, Bundy AC (Eds). *Sensory Integration: Theory and Practice*. Philadelphia: Davis. pp. 92–9.

Fisher AG, Murray EA, Bundy AC (1991) *Sensory Integration: Theory and Practice*. Philadelphia: Davis.

Forssberg H, Nashner LM (1982) Cited in Richardson PK, Atwater SW, Crowe TK, Deitz JC (1992) Performance of preschoolers on the Pediatric Clinical Test of Sensory Interaction for Balance. *American Journal of Occupational Therapy* 46(9): 793–800.

Foster M (1996) in Turner A, Foster M, Johnson SE, *Occupational Therapy and Physical Dysfunction Principles, Skills and Practice*. New York: Churchill Livingstone.

Gallahue DL (1976) *Motor Development and Movement Experiences for Young Children*. St Louis: Mosby.

Gardner MF (1988) *Test of Visual Perceptual Skills (Non-motor)*. Burlingame: Psychological and Educational Publications.

Golden CJ, Hemmeke TA, Purisch AD (1980) *The Luria–Nebraska Neuropsychological Battery: Children's Revision*. Los Angeles: Western Psychological Services.

Goodenough FL, Harris DB (1963) *Goodenough–Harris Drawing Test*. Los Angeles: Western Psychological Services.

Hagedorn R (1995) *Occupational Therapy: Perspectives and Processes*. Edinburgh: Churchill Livingstone.

Hammill DD, Bryant BR (1986) *Detroit Tests of Learning Aptitude–Primary*. Austin TX: Pro-Ed.

Hammill DD, Pearson NA, Voress JK (1993) *Developmental Test of Visual Perception – 2*, Austin TX: Pro-Ed.

Haradon G, Bascom B, Dragomir C, Scripcaru V (1994) Sensory functions of institutionalised Romanian infants: a pilot study. *Occupational Therapy International* 1: 250–60.

Hattie J, Edwards H (1987) A review of the Bruininks–Oseretsky test of motor proficiency. *British Journal of Educational Psychology* 57: 104–113.

Hayes SC, Nelson RO, Jarrett RB (1987) The treatment utility of assessment: a functional approach to evaluating assessment quality. *American Psychologist* 42(11): 963–74.

Henderson SE, Sugden DA (1992) *The Movement Assessment Battery for Children*. London: Psychological Corporation.

Howard L (1997) Developmental coordination disorder: can we measure our intervention? *British Journal of Occupational Therapy* 60(5): 219–20.

Hummell J (1980) *Sensory Motor Processes. Part III: History*. Unpublished class notes, Cumberland College of Health Sciences, University of Sydney.

Irlen H (1991) *Reading by the Colours: Overcoming Dyslexia and Other Reading Disabilities Through the Irlen Method*. New York: Avery.

Johnson J (1977) Cited in Wilson B, Pollock N, Kaplan BJ, Law M, Faris P (1992) Reliability and construct validity of the clinical observations of motor and postural skills. *American Journal of Occupational Therapy* 46(9): 775–83.

Kaufman AS, Kaufman NL (1983) *Kaufman Assessment Battery for Children*. Circle Pines: American Guidance Service.

Kimball JG (1990) Using the sensory integration and praxis test to measure change: a pilot study. *American Journal of Occupational Therapy* 44(7): 603–8.

Kirk SA, Gallagher JJ (1983) Cited in American Occupational Therapy Association (1991) Statement: Occupational therapy provision for children with learning disabilities and/or mild to moderate perceptual and motor deficits. *American Journal of Occupational Therapy* 45(12): 1069–74.

Koppitz EM (1975) *Bender Gestalt Test for Young Children. Volume II: Research and Application 1963–1973*. New York: Grune and Stratton.

Lai JS, Fisher AG, Magathaes LC, Bundy AC (1996) Construct validity of the sensory integration and praxis test. *Occupational Therapy Journal of Research* 16(2): 75–97.

Lambert NM (1988) Cited in Farley SK, Sarracino T, Howard PM (1991) Development of a treatment rating in school systems: service determination through objective measurement. *American Journal of Occupational Therapy* 45(10): 898–906.

Leonardelli Haertlein CA (1992) Ethics in evaluation in occupational therapy. *American Journal of Occupational Therapy* 46(10): 950–3.

Lerner J (1985) Cited in American Occupational Therapy Association (1991) Statement: Occupational therapy provision for children with learning disabilities and/or mild to moderate perceptual and motor deficits. *American Journal of Occupational Therapy* 45(12): 1069–74.

Levine MD (1993) *Developmental Variation and Learning Disorders*. Cambridge: Education.

Losse A, Henderson S, Elliman D Hall D, Knight E, Jongmans M (1991) Clumsiness in children – do they grow out of it? A 10 year follow up study. *Developmental Medicine and Child Neurology* 33: 55–68.

Lunz ME, Stahl JA (1990) Cited in Wilson B, Pollock N, Kaplan BJ, Law M, Faris P (1992) Reliability and construct validity of the clinical observations of motor and postural skills. *American Journal of Occupational Therapy* 46(9):775–83.

McCarron LT (1982) *McCarron Assessment of Neuromuscular Development*. Dallas: Common Market Press.

McConnell D (1993) *Clinical Observations and Clumsy Children: Is There a Relationship?* Unpublished Honours thesis, Cumberland College of Health Sciences. University of Sydney.

McConnell DB (1994) Clinical observations and developmental coordination disorders. Is there a relationship? *Occupational Therapy International* 1: 278–91.

McLoughlin JA, Lewis RB (1986) *Assessing Special Students*. Columbus: Merrill.

Magalhaes LC, Koomar, JA, Cermak SA (1989) Bilateral motor coordination in 5 to 9 year old children: a pilot study, *American Journal of Occupational Therapy* 43(7): 437 43.

Michael WB (1985) Review of Miller assessment for preschoolers. In Mitchell JV (Ed). *The Ninth Mental Measurements Yearbook*. Lincoln: University of Nebraska Press.

Miller LJ (1988a) cited in American Occupational Therapy Association (1991) Statement: Occupational therapy provision for children with learning disabilities and/or mild to moderate perceptual and motor deficits. *American Journal of Occupational Therapy* 45(12): 1069–74.

Miller LJ (1988b) *Miller Assessment for Preschoolers: Manual*. Revised edn. San Antonio: Psychological Corporation.

Miller LJ (1988c) *Miller Assessment for Preschoolers: Seminar, Administration and Interpretation*. San Antonio: Psychological Corporation.

Miller LJ (1990) *Overview of Other Scales for Assessing Preschoolers*. Englewood: KID Foundation.

Miller LJ (1992) *The Screening Test for Evaluating Preschoolers (First STEP)* Englewood: KID Foundation.

Miller LJ (1993a) *The Infant/Toddler Screening for Everybaby (ITSE)*. Englewood: KID Foundation.

Miller LJ (1993b) *The Miller Toddler and Infant Evaluation (TIME)*. Tucson: Therapy Skills Builders.

Mooti, Sterling, Spalding (1978) Quick Neurological Screening Test. Cited in Wilson B, Pollock N, Kaplan BJ, Law M, Faris P (1996) Reliability and construct validity of the clinical observations of motor and postural skills. *American Journal of Occupational Therapy* 46(9): 775–83.

Moryosef-Ittah S, Hinojosa J (1992b) Discriminant validity of the Developmental Test of Visual Perception–2 for children with learning disabilities. *Occupational Therapy International* 3(3): 204–11.

Murray EA, Cermak SA, O'Brien V (1990) The relationship between form and space perception, constructional abilities, and clumsiness in children. *American Journal of Occupational Therapy* 44(7): 623–8.

Northern Territory Department of Education (1990) *Early Childhood Education Preschool to Year 3 Screening and Assessment*. Darwin: Northern Territory Department of Education.

Oliver CE (1990) A sensorimotor program for improving writing readiness skills in elementary-age children. *American Journal of Occupational Therapy* 44(2): 111–6.

Ottenbacher K, Short A, Watson PJ (1979) Nystagmus duration changes of learning disabled children during sensory integrative therapy. *Perceptual Motor Skills* 48: 1159 –64.

Parham LD (1990) Is sensory integration related to achievement? A longitudinal study of elementary school children. *Sensory Integration Quarterly* March: 9, 16.

Parham, LD (1996) Perspectives on play. In Zemke R, Clark F (1996) *Occupational Science – the Evolving Discipline*. Philadelphia: Davis FA.

Phillips RC (1976) *The Skills of Handwriting*. Oxford: Phillips.

Pickard P, Alston J (1985) *Helping Secondary School Pupils with Handwriting: Current Research, Identification and Assessment, Guidance*. Wisbech: LDA.

Piers EV, Harris DB (1984) *The Piers–Harris Childrens Self-concept Scale: Revised Manual*. Los Angeles: Western Psychological Services.

Richardson PK, Atwater SW, Crowe TK, Deitz JC (1992) Performance of preschoolers on the Pediatric Clinical Test of Sensory Interaction for Balance. *American Journal of Occupational Therapy* 46(9): 793–800.

Royeen CB, Fortune JC (1990) Touch inventory for elementary school-aged children. *American Journal of Occupational Therapy* 44: 165–170.

Salvia J, Ysseldyke JE (1991) *Assessment*. Boston: Houghton Mifflin.

Shoemaker M, Hijlkema M, Kalverboer A (1994) Physiotherapy for clumsy children: an evaluation study. *Developmental Medicine and Child Neurology* 36: 143–55.

Short-DeGraff MA, Holan S (1992) Self-drawing as a gauge of perceptual–motor skill. *Physical and Occupational Therapy in Pediatrics* 12(1): 53–68.

Smith CR (1983) Cited in American Occupational Therapy Association (1991) Statement: Occupational therapy provision for children with learning disabilities and/or mild to moderate perceptual and motor deficits. *American Journal of Occupational Therapy* 45(12): 1069–74.

Stallings-Sahler S (1990) Report of an occupational therapy evaluation of sensory integration and praxis. *American Journal of Occupational Therapy* 44(7): 650–3.

Stott DH, Moyes FA, Henderson SE (1985) *Diagnosis and Remediation of Handwriting Problems.* Guelph: Brook Educational.

Stott DH, Moyes FA, Henderson SE (1989) *Test of Motor Impairment.* San Antonio: Psychological Corporation.

Tseng MH, Murray EA (1994) Differences in Perceptual–Motor Measures in Children with Good and Poor Handwriting. *Occupational Therapy Journal of Research* 14(1): 19–36.

Vaugh S, Lyon GR (1994) Ethical considerations when conducting research with students with learning disabilities. In Vaugh S, Bos CS (1994) *Research Issues in Learning Disabilities: Theory, Methodology, Assessment and Ethics.* New York: Springer-Vergag.

Wilson BN, Kaplan BJ, Fellowes S, Gruchy C, Faris P (1992a) The efficacy of sensory integration treatment compared to tutoring. *Physical and Occupational Therapy in Pediatrics* 12(1): 1–36.

Wilson BN, Pollock N, Kaplan BJ, Law M, Faris P (1992b) Reliability and construct validity of the clinical observations of motor and postural skills. *American Journal of Occupational Therapy* 46(9): 775–83.

Wilson B, Pollock N, Kaplan B, Law M (1994) *Clinical Observations of Motor and Postural Skills (COMPS).* San Antonio: Psychological Corporation.

Wilson EB (1984) *Occupational Therapy for Children with Minimal Handicaps.* Unpublished manual.

Wiss T, Clark F (1990) Validity of the Southern California Postrotary Nystagmus Test: misconceptions lead to incorrect conclusions. *American Journal of Occupational Therapy* 44(7): 658–60.

Yack E (1989) Sensory integration: a survey of its use in the clinical setting. *Canadian Journal of Occupational Therapy* 56(5): 229–35.

Ziviani J, Elkin J (1984) An evaluation of handwriting performance. *Educational Review* 36:3.

Ziviani J, Elkin J (1986) Effect of pencil grip on handwriting speed and legibility. *Educational Review* 38:247–57.

Ziviani J, Poulsen A, O'Brien A (1982) Correlation of the Bruininks–Oseretsky test of motor proficiency with the Southern California Sensory Integration Tests. *American Journal of Occupational Therapy* 36: 519–23.

Ziviani J, Hayes A, Chant D (1990) Handwriting: a perceptual motor disturbance in children with myelomeningocele. *Occupational Therapy Journal of Research* 10: 12–26.

Chapter 3
The Treatment Session

Elaine B. Wilson

The therapy session is an enjoyable experience for both you and the child. However, you will soon realise that no two children have exactly the same problems, although the experience that you gain with each child can help you to select the appropriate treatment. You will probably need to change the combinations of methods that you use as treatment progresses. At times, a totally different approach is needed, for example, to deal with parents' problems, or with a variation from the original treatment plan should a child's behaviour be unacceptable. Although a core of basic methods is available and many children have similar deficits, there really are no absolute rules. Be prepared for anything, either at the time of the initial assessment or at any stage throughout treatment, and adjust the plan accordingly.

Ensure that activities are age appropriate. For example, where you might use a stuffed toy with a young child, you would use a sand bag/ball for someone older.

Above all, remember that for the treatment to be fully beneficial, it must be **fun** for children. If it is not fun, do not treat in that way; work out another way to make the session enjoyable. Any possible benefit from forced treatment will be negated by the resistance to participate.

How many children can you treat at once?

The essence of an effective programme is to balance the challenge of the task against the child's ability to achieve it. This will involve the child in working hard, showing initiative and obviously enjoying the process. Simultaneously, the therapist provides positive support but does not directly intervene to manipulate the child or the task (Tickle-Degman and Coster, 1995, p. 122).

Many therapists find that they need to work on a one-to-one basis to individualise the intervention (Fisher *et al.*, 1991). However, some find that they can treat two children at once, without help, although it can be very difficult. Preferably, either an assistant or a parent should help. If possible, treat two children who are of the same sex and similar age and size. It is usually more fun for the children and they give each other courage to try new activities. It is also more cost-effective. If the two children selected to have therapy together are not compatible, change one for another more suitable child. Treat individually a child whose behaviour is so poor that it would distract another child or who would be distracted by a second child.

If there are several assistants, you can treat six to eight younger (pre-school age) children in a group, but a more structured programme is needed. Using groups of four to six school-aged children can be very successful. Both these situations can also reduce long waiting lists. Have the school-aged sessions twice weekly for $1\frac{1}{2}$ hours for a period of six weeks (for example during the long school holidays). One therapist or assistant is needed for every two children. Base your decision about how many children to treat at once on your experience, on the individual needs of the child, on the help you can enlist, on the space and equipment that are available and on what you personally feel able to manage. Official or unofficial parent support groups can form as a result of these group sessions.

Some centres set up treatment stations when working with groups of school-aged children. Sellers (1989), for example, had eight stations (perceptual motor, physical fitness, rhythm, balance, manipulation, body awareness and stunts, loco-motor and fine motor/visual motor activities). The children attended twice weekly for 45 minutes each session. The staff ratio was ideally one-to-one or one-to-two. The amount of time each child spent at a station depended on the child's attention span and interest. Most spent approximately 10 minutes on each and would thus not visit all stations in one session.

Blocks of treatment

The author typically treats children in blocks of approximately 12 sessions. Some British occupational therapists have found that eight sessions are sufficient; others offer more. The decision has to be based on effective progress or outcomes (McDerment, personal communication, 1997).

Plan each session to take 55 minutes and spend five minutes at the end of the session writing a brief report on each child seen. Remind the parents of the plan so that they will not feel that their child is being 'rejected' when the block of treatment ends.

Most children are ready to cease after 12 sessions; this readiness may manifest as indifference, lack of interest, bored looks or unwillingness to attend the session. Frequently, and often without warning, these behaviour patterns appear as the block of therapy sessions draws to a close. Reassess the child with some of the original non-standardised tests at about week eight in order to determine how many deficits still need correcting; then concentrate your efforts on these areas.

If, after 12 sessions, the child is still enjoying therapy and some deficits remain, continue therapy for four to six more sessions. Children rarely benefit fully from treatment until it ceases – integration continues and usually becomes more efficiently processed later. Some children benefit from having a break of four to six weeks. After such a break, resume and concentrate on the one or two remaining deficits.

A card system is useful. Highlight each child's current treatment aims on the left hand side of the front of a card to which you can easily refer. Use the right side of the card for notes, for example, the child's low tolerance to movement, gravitational insecurity or tactile defensiveness, or to record the loan of a book to a parent. Write brief daily reports on the back of the card or in progress notes, i.e. whichever system is in place in the department.

Regression effects

During the first session, warn the parents about regression effects, such as nausea (or vomiting), overactivity, aggression towards other children immediately after the therapy session, headache, irritability, tearfulness, excessive tiredness or deterioration in schoolwork, that may follow therapy. Ask the parents to contact you immediately if the regression effects are distressing for the child, or report them at the next session if the effects are minor. Stress that these effects are not common, but all parents need to be warned so that they are not concerned if they occur.

The author has found that regression effects may follow treatment sessions immediately, a day or so later (in the case of delayed vestibular effects) or occasionally several weeks later, perhaps through a build-up of stimulation to the nervous system or even its overstimulation or disorganisation. Do not confuse these regression effects with the normal development of assertiveness in the formerly timid child. Assertiveness can be a very positive result of treatment; reassure parents that these changes are good for the child. Modify the treatment programme to prevent the effects recurring. For example, give the child few vestibular-proprioceptive activities, take longer to calm him at the end of treatment and/or provide him with fewer overall stimulating activities.

Precautions

- Under no circumstances, take any risks.
- Check equipment for wear at least every six months. Check ceiling attachments and have them inspected by qualified maintenance staff every six months or when they begin to show the slightest sign of unsafe wear. Check ropes for fraying; replace any worn ropes or metal-on-metal attachments.
- Check that the child's placement on or in the equipment is correct before he begins the activity. Never leave a child unattended or unwatched. Consider taking out extra professional liability insurance to cover situations that could result in injury.
- Do not let the child use the scooter board as a skateboard.
- Watch for any of the following negative signs and symptoms from the activities: nausea, pallor, sweating, redness, shortness of breath and drowsiness. If these signs occur, do not panic but change immediately to a calming activity. For

example, some children enjoy being massaged by a vibrator while they lie in a bean bag.

- Observe the child's overt and covert reactions and discontinue any activity that the child wants to stop. When you provide the input, you impose that input and the child has no control over it, in contrast to the child's self-activation with the activity.
- When you administer sensory integrative treatment procedures to children who have ventricle shunts, avoid fast vestibular activities in the first few sessions. Treat the child in an upright position. If no adverse effects are reported, you can be more adventurous and provide activities in other positions, for example on the hands and knees, lying or rolling.
- When you treat children who experience controlled or uncontrolled seizures, avoid rotary vestibular activities because such activities can cause hyperventilation. Activities to avoid include jumping up and down on a tractor inner tube or fast movement in a net hammock. Also avoid any activity where there is a quick change of light and shadow, such as looking out into bright sunlight and then looking inside at the darker wall. If you use a hammock with these children, ensure that the speed is slow and rhythmical. Alternatively, you could encourage linear, between two suspension points, rather than rotary stimulation.

Positive reinforcers

For some children, the enjoyment of sessions and achievement is enough reinforcement. However, if felt appropriate, a reinforcer in the treatment session needs to be only very simple. It may be verbal praise along with a star on a cardboard chart, a star on the board for that day, a stamp on the hand, a choice for the next activity or even a hug. The child must want that reinforcer so that he will work for it. Parents can use the same principles. They can use a star chart placed on the fridge, with a column for each day. There must be the same contract principles whereby the parents state what they want their child to do, and they must discuss with him what he wants as the (realistic) reward. If the child does not want the reward, he will not work for it; always gear this towards the child by finding individual motivators.

Difficulties that may arise in any treatment session

During a treatment session (or later), a child may display atypical behaviour. He may run around, hide, become hyperactive, tearful or uncooperative, or be totally out of control. If this occurs, stop the treatment and deal with the change in behaviour that results from the apparent 'disorganisation'.

Management of behaviour in the treatment session

You will also encounter a child who will 'test' you and misbehave. All his life he has failed, and, in order to survive, he has tested and manipulated people – usually his mother in particular. It is essential to identify whether aberrant behaviour occurs at school, at home, socially/at sport or just in treatment sessions. Identify whether different problems are arising in different settings. The child who tests you is usually one whose parents report difficulty with their child's behaviour, so they can use the same principles as you. For the child who behaves in this way, you are advised to:

- treat him or her singly
- request the mother/parents/carer not to stay for the therapy session if his behaviour is worse in their presence
- be hard on the problem and soft on the person.

The following suggestions are for the children who are continually testing you or who are misbehaving because that is the way they work. The suggestions can also be used for the children whose nervous system has become 'disorganised' as a result of treatment or overstimulation, although use the principles of calming and management (see pp. 63–6) for that time.

Canter and Canter (1988) have suggested some basics for management of behaviour, as outlined below.

1. You are the boss (of your department)

Once the child knows this, it is much easier. If, within reason, he does not comply, look him in the eye and calmly say, for example, 'I want you to lie on the scooter board, and I will pull you around' or 'You and I are going to ride on the bolster swing.'

Repeat and repeat and repeat, like a broken record. Stand firm with your request. **Give positive reinforcement when he complies**.

2. Be consistent

Consistency is the key to effective management. If you state the behaviour you want, you must maintain that decision: 'You can have a swing in the net after you have jumped on the mini-trampoline and hit the ball *straight* to me 20 times.' **Give positive reinforcement when he complies**.

3. Create structure

Involve him in a 'contract' – work out, together, a *structured* plan of treatment for the rest of the session (and future sessions if this behaviour is common) and ask the child to write it on the board. If the child is not old enough to write, he or you can draw pictures of the activities planned. Let the child choose one – it must be appropriate – then you choose one and so on. You may elect to allow him to choose all the activities, with some monitoring from you. He is far more likely to adhere to the list and comply with what is set out. Jordan (1988) also suggests giving a child light structure and having consistent discipline.

4. Set physical and verbal boundaries

These are a few examples:

- have the child on the bolster swing and sit closely behind him, or
- have him in the corner of the room and bounce a ball back and forth to him, or
- put him in the barrel on the scooter board and pull him around, or
- meet him at the bottom of the ramp after he goes down. Take his hand and bring him back to the top of the ramp. Keep repeating this procedure, or
- tell him you want him to jump on the tractor inner tube for 20 jumps and then stop. When he does this, you say 'Stop' and make sure he does *totally* stop. Repeat this a few times.
  Give positive reinforcement when he complies.

If he runs away, make sure that all the doors are locked so that the child cannot endanger himself outside, but do not chase him. His safety must be paramount, and he must not have access to the road and its traffic because he is likely to be out of control and act without thought. If he is safely in the room, pretend to ignore him; do some other task.

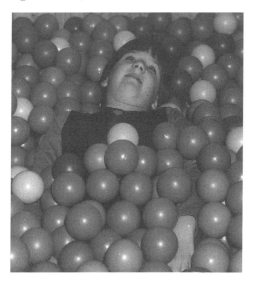

Figure 3.1: Lying in a box of balls

Time out

If a child gets out of control, it is good to have some equipment on the floor that he can have 'time out' in or on:

- a deep box, one third full with foam pellets that he can get into; a large box of balls (Fig 3.1) that he can get into and hide
- a soft rubber mat to stand on, or an upturned box to sit on with the soft rubber mat placed on top of it (Fig 3.2)

- a square piece of fur fabric that the child can lie on
- a plastic hoop that he can stand in
- a piece of cardboard with feet painted on it that he can put his own feet on top of
- while he is on or in the above, you can elect to incorporate an interesting fine motor or fine visual space activity or, for example, play a game of mazes or 'boxes' on the blackboard or whiteboard.

These physical boundaries can have an incredibly sobering effect on a child, see Figure 3.3. Often just the mere 'threat' of going onto or into 'time out' equipment will result in more self-control. **When he is in control, give him positive reinforcement.**

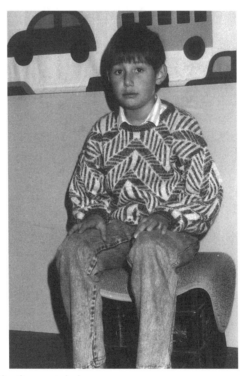

Figure 3.2: Sitting on the time-out chair

Temper tantrums at home

The above principles can also be used at home. French (personal communication 1993) suggests a piece of cardboard with the child's own feet drawn on it and placed in his bedroom. This is good because he can go into his bedroom and jump up and down for a short time when he feels angry. She also suggests that the parents have an onion or orange sack filled with foam or a sheet, suspended from a tree in the back garden, this can be the child's punch-bag.

Whatever situation is presented, ranging from overactivity to being completely out of control, allow the child to earn the right to start again, as Joanna Nicklin states in Chapter 4, but thereafter keep to calming activities for the rest of the session. You must forgive and allow him to try again.

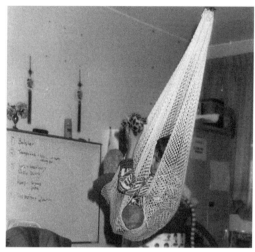

Figure 3.3: Physical boundaries of a net together with slow rotary movement can help to calm the child

The parents can use the above principles for managing their child at home. Encourage them to tell you about the problems they are having with their child and discuss with them some management strategies. It is also essential that they communicate with each other and with the teachers, and always work as a team. A book is a good means of communicating progress and reporting between teachers and parents; this keeps everyone informed of what is happening. It is a good method to monitor behaviour, particularly if children commence medication or undergo the food challenge (see Appendix 5). With teamwork, the child realises that his manipulative techniques are not effective.

It is good advice for parents to reinforce their children's behaviour; every day, they must find three things that can be positively reinforced. The results, for all concerned, can be most rewarding.

Parents' role in therapy

Parents usually attend and assist in the session; they like to be involved and to know what is happening during therapy. The therapist should always provide explanatory handouts for parents, and for parents to give to the child's teacher. This sets up a two-way communication system between the therapist and the teacher. A 'parents' night' with a group of families, teachers and friends can be very beneficial for reinforcing the rationale behind therapy and treatment procedures. Show a short video of treatment if you have one because the other parent or teacher who is not at the treatment sessions often does not understand the concept behind it. The therapy video removes anxiety about what is happening to the child. Emphasise to the parents the importance of treating their children 'normally'. At supper-time – it is *essential* to have supper – parents and friends can talk to you and to each other.

During the first session, discuss the treatment plan with the parents and child. Outline the likely duration of treatment and explain that most children are ready for a break after that period. Ask the parents to observe the child closely during the week between sessions. In this first session, you must warn the parents of regression effects from treatment (see p. 34).

At the beginning of each session (or at another convenient point), ask the parent about the child's progress and establish whether or not any problems have arisen. If necessary, suggest approaches that the parents can use to overcome problems and to reinforce advances made during sessions. During each session, discuss the child's progress and improvements with the parents and explain your plans for improving the weak areas. Be selective as to whether or not you do this in front of the child.

After two or three sessions, when you have evaluated the child's reaction to treatment, suggest a home programme (see Appendix 3) involving one or two activities that the child likes and that the parents can supervise; a number of parents also ask to be able to carry over some activities at home. The home programme reinforces the work of the weekly sessions. If the home programme causes problems for either child or parents, advise the parents to stop it. If it is apparent that the child–parent relationship is strained, you may choose not to mention the home programme.

In preparing the home programme, assess the demands being made on the mother or father and design a home programme that is both realistic and supportive:

- Are both parents working?
- Are their working hours regular or do they change (e.g. shiftwork)?
- How many other children are in the family, and what are their ages?
- Will the parent(s) or another relative make or erect any equipment that is required?
- What are the parents/carers already doing with the child?

Try to assess the parents' coping skills as well as their attitude towards their child's need for therapy; do not overload parents who already are at their limits. As well as these factors, the child may have a very tiring day, for example, travelling long distances in the school bus. It should be remembered, however, that *any* related activities done at home are usually better than none.

Treatment session

Although it may be your practice to treat one child at a time, the following descriptions of activities assume that you are (hypothetically) treating two children together and that at least one person assists you. **Even though the complete range of activities is described, you will select activities to meet the needs identified during the assessment.**

Ask all children to remove their shoes and socks. Most will agree to do so, but children who object firmly are usually tactually defensive or have not mastered the skill. Do not insist that these children comply.

To reinforce the motor planning of an activity, ask the child to describe, before the activity, what he is going to do. When it is completed, ask him for feedback on the success of what he has just done.

In session one, orientate the child to the clinic and equipment. Put the child on each piece of equipment briefly to let him get the 'feel' of the activities. Observe the child's reaction and behaviour. If the child is initially very resistant, it may even be necessary for the mother to do the treating under your instruction. Timid or very compliant children will sometimes say nothing (to you) during the session but may report to parents that certain equipment was good fun or awful. Ask the parents to tell you the child's responses at the next session. This orientation to the activities is vital. In subsequent sessions, follow the treatment plan that you developed after you assessed the child. Where possible, let the child initiate the activity – he will often be keen to explore the new environment, so involve him in activity selection.

Bolster swing – linear movement

Commence with linear movement. Have the children sit on the bolster swing and catch beanbags in a sand bucket, catch a toy animal in one hand and throw it across their body's midline into a receptacle, or catch balls in the game of Grip ball. After two or three minutes, have the children lie prone on the bolster and hug it tightly (Fig 3.4). Swing them vigorously for two or three minutes to make it challenging. Repeat these activities with the children in the kneeling, half-kneeling (Fig 3.5) and standing positions (allowing two or three minutes in each position). Even pre-school children can usually manage to stand on the moving bolster. Watch for

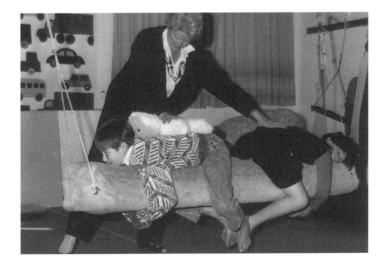

Figure 3.4: Hugging a bolster swing

signs of gravitational insecurity, such as a look of fear on the child's face or a comment such as 'Don't go too fast'. Ask gravitationally insecure children to move the bolster swing themselves: say, 'You be the driver.' Alternatively, if a child is very insecure on the bolster in early sessions, you may get on it with him. Maybe talk about 'riding the horse' together. Sitting in the centre of the bolster, provides additional proprioceptive input and balance (Fig 3.6). A child sitting alone in the centre of the bolster can push it back and forth himself using a long broom handle. He is then 'paddling his canoe' and crossing the midline as he 'paddles' either side of the bolster (Fig 3.7).

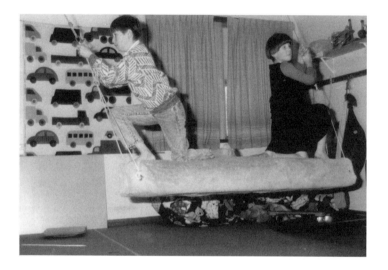

Figure 3.5: Half-kneeling on a bolster

Dual swing – rotary movement

Place the children into a dual swing ('helicopter'), the children putting their legs into the loops and holding the ropes. With help from an assistant, hold the children out and set them moving (Fig 3.8). Change direction every 30 seconds by grabbing each child and stopping him quickly. If the children are of different sizes, the small child will orbit out, while the heavier one stays down. It is better then to have both children going around together, against each other, one child in front of the other (Fig 3.9). If only one child is in the dual swing, hold onto the other loops and swing her around (Fig 3.10); change direction as mentioned above. Watch the children's reactions. If one child is not enjoying this activity, stop it immediately. Remember that although they are directing you, they do not control the movement.

Alternate linear and rotary vestibular-proprioceptive activities to provide variety. Some children cannot tolerate rotary movement for longer than two or three minutes but will tolerate linear movement for longer, even though all parts of the vestibular apparatus fire signals continuously.

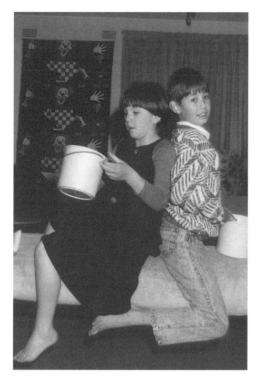
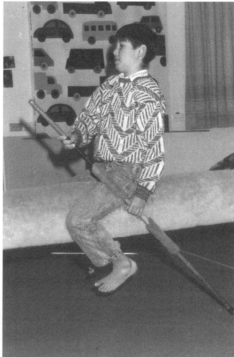

Figure 3.6: Sitting back-to-back on a bolster   **Figure 3.7:** 'Paddling a canoe' on a bolster

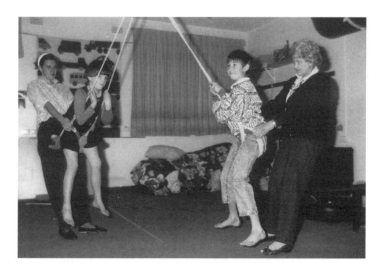

Figure 3.8: Holding children in a dual swing

Ramp – prone extension, supine flexion postures, balance

First, have each child prone on a scooter board at the top of the ramp. Facilitate a prone extension posture by placing a toy animal on the back of the child's thighs to keep them together (Fig 3.11). For an older child, a small beanbag or sand bag can be used. Tell the child, 'You must not drop the [named] animal/bag'. If the child's legs still do not stay together, place a 50 mm circular strip of inner tube (made by cutting across the tube) around the child's thighs or knees. If the child does not assume a good prone extension posture, or if he flexes his hips when you ask him to extend his head and hips, hold his legs up, extend them from the hips and press on the back of his head (Fig 3.12). This will help him to understand the posture required, and he will automatically assume the posture before he 'scoots' down the ramp (Fig 3.13). It may be necessary to demonstrate that position a few times.

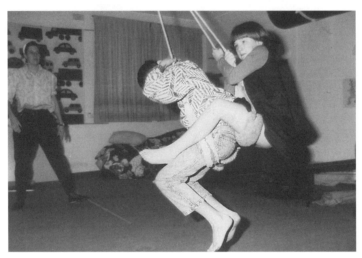

Figure 3.9: Swinging around together in a dual swing

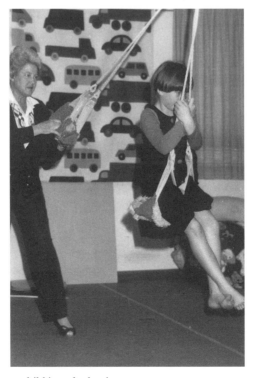

Figure 3.10: Swinging one child in a dual swing

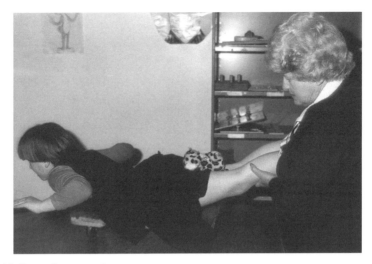

Figure 3.11: Preparing to go down a ramp

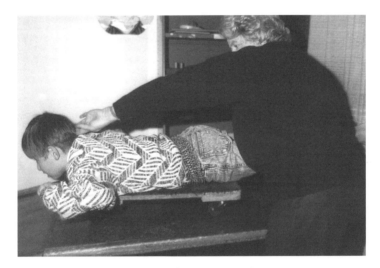

Figure 3.12: Pressing on the child's head to facilitate extension

Grasp the child's thighs, move him on the board to the edge of the ramp and launch him. Instruct him to catch an animal (Fig 3.14) or hit a soft ball suspended overhead as he goes down. Repeat this activity no more than three times and then have the child assume the supine flexed position on the board. The child lies on the scooter board, flexes his knees, hips and neck, and brings his head up. Say, 'Look at Mum' (who is standing at the bottom of the ramp) so that the child will correctly assume the supine flexed position. Launch the child and instruct him to catch a toy animal or a soft ball between his legs (Fig 3.15). Repeat this activity three times.

Next, have the child sit and then kneel; begin with low knees (squatting on her heels), then move to upright knees (Fig 3.16) and then to kneeling with the arms held high above her head. This activity raises the centre of gravity and challenges the child. Hold her lower legs together on the scooter board as she goes over the ridge of the ramp until she starts to scoot down the ramp. Instruct her to catch a ball or animal as she descends.

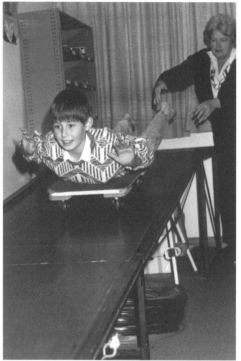

Figure 3.13: Scooting down a ramp

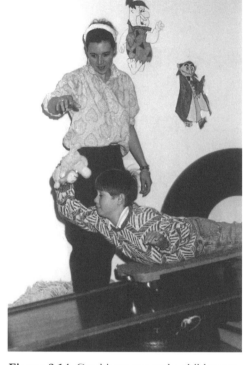

Figure 3.14: Catching a toy as the child scoots down a ramp

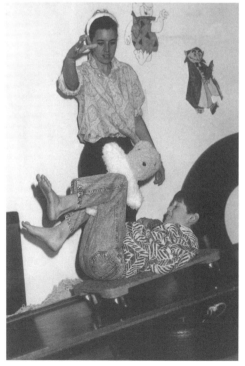

Figure 3.15: Catching a toy as the child goes down supine

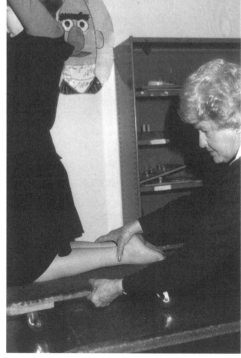

Figure 3.16: Launching the child down a ramp on upright knees

A final upgrade is the 'Captain Cook' posture (which the children enjoy). In this, the child scoots down the ramp with one foot on the scooter board, one knee on it and one hand on his forehead ('looking out for land') (Fig 3.17). It is usually too hard to balance and catch anything in this position, so the activity is just to assume the challenging posture. With any ramp work, you can move the child on the scooter board in several directions at the top of the ramp before you launch him, giving him extra sensory input.

Horizontal tyre – rotary movement

Sit two children on the tyre and swing the tyre around fairly gently (Fig 3.18), changing the direction of movement every 30 seconds. Place a large sheet of cardboard on the floor. Throw a beanbag for the child to catch and ask him to throw it onto a letter drawn on the cardboard sheet. Then ask the child to think of a word that begins with that letter. Match the difficulty with the children's ability.

Alternatively, have the children throw beanbags onto a sheet of cardboard with pictures on and ask the children to describe the pictures. Children greatly enjoy this activity, and it is good for those who have a low tolerance to movement or who have speech problems. If a child lies across the tyre, in a prone extension position (Fig 3.19) or through it (Fig 3.20), leaning on the tyre to run back and forth, place a sheepskin over the rubber to make it more comfortable.

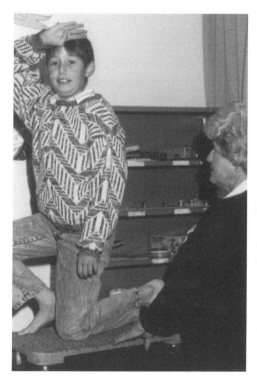

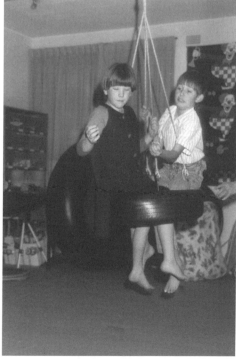

Figure 3.17: Assuming the 'Captain Cook' posture

Figure 3.18: Swinging in a horizontal tyre

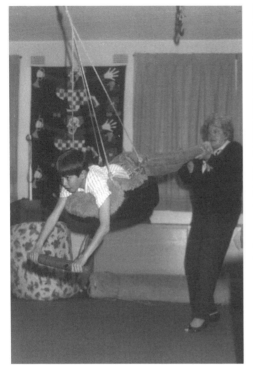
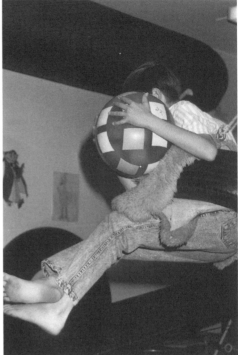

Figure 3.19: Lying prone on a horizontal tyre   **Figure 3.20:** Lying through a horizontal tyre

Jumping on mini-trampolines while hitting balls – bilateral and linear vestibular activity

Align the mini-trampolines and have each child stand on one holding a rolling pin or broomstick covered with materials of different texture, using both hands (to improve bilateral function). Stand five or six metres away from the children and bounce the balls to them as they rebound on the trampoline. They must hit down with the rolling pin as they jump so that bilateral function is obtained; the balls are also easier to catch and you run around less! Begin by throwing balls directly to the child, initially using a large inflated beach ball and then decreasing the ball diameters. If you work with an assistant, simultaneously bounce the balls to the child *diagonally* opposite you – this is fun for children, especially when the balls hit each other! Remember to use balls that bounce well and, if possible, try them out on *your* own therapy room or similar floor surface before you purchase them.

Similar activities can also be carried out on a normal-sized trampoline.

Flexor swing – rotary movement with eye–hand co-ordination

Have one child stand and the other sit on the platform of the swing and 'hug' the central piece. Move the swing back, forth and round while your assistant throws soft toy animals or beanbags to the children. Instruct them to catch and throw the articles into a receptacle: a cane hoop, a tractor inner tube, a barrel or five inner tubes. Adjust the location and size of the receptacles according to the children's ages and capabilities. After about six minutes, swap the children's positions or, alternatively, have both children stand or sit. Because this activity involves extensive eye–hand co-ordination, which can be inhibitory, it is good for children who have low vestibular tolerance. Teenagers also enjoy the activity, and it can be made quite challenging by throwing the article in all directions for them to catch it.

Tractor inner tube – increasing muscle tone, balance

Have the children straddle and bounce around on the tube and change directions when you call (Fig 3.21). Alternatively, they can stand on the tube and play a game of 'traffic lights' using three coloured balls or coloured circle cards – red (stop), orange (go slowly) and green (go fast). Hold up one ball or card at a time and instruct the children to move according to its colour.

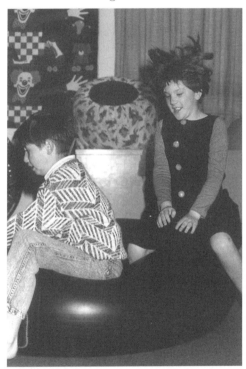

Figure 3.21: Bouncing on a tractor inner tube

You can also have the children walk quickly around the inner tube and catch a ball or just stand on the tube and hit the ball down with a rolling pin or broomstick, as described for the activity with mini-trampolines.

Alternatively, you can hold onto the child's hands and allow her to jump on the tractor inner tube (Fig 3.22). If the tube is not sufficiently stable while the child bounces, put a small amount of water in it or place one of your feet under the tube (Fig 3.23) to stabilise it.

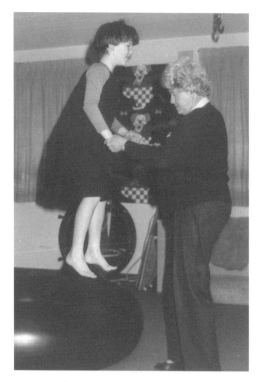

Figure 3.22: Jumping on a tractor inner tube

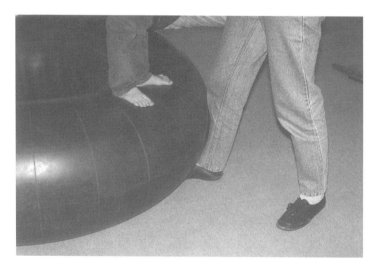

Figure 3.23: Stabilising a tractor inner tube with the foot

Rolling in a barrel or a set of five inner tubes – rotary vestibular activity

Have one child lie in the car inner tubes and another child lie in the large barrel turned on its side (Fig 3.24). With one child at each end of the room, ask the children to roll towards each other and 'crash'. Then have them return to the ends of the room and come together again. Encourage them to roll themselves, rather than rolling them yourself, because active rolling is more integrating. Some children will, however, need assistance because this activity is physically demanding.

You can also get the child to pick up a beanbag or quoit and roll across the room, put it in a box or on a peg and then go back and repeat the activity. If working with an individual child, the time taken can be recorded; in the next session the child can then be encouraged to go faster. If working in pairs, you can make it a race.

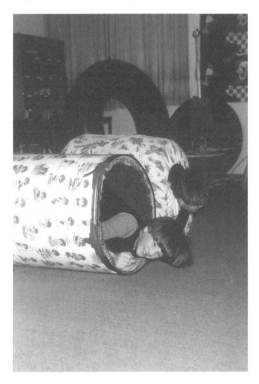

Figure 3.24: Rolling in a barrel and five inner tubes

Prone in a net or dual swing – linear movement

Place one child prone in the net as follows. Hold the net out so the child can put one knee into it and then the other. Then the child places his hands on your shoulders and 'flops down' (Fig 3.25). Tie him in, above his neck or upper trunk (Fig 3.26). Place the other child in the dual swing in the 'Superman' position (Fig 3.27), with each arm and leg in a loop. Facilitate the prone extension posture while the children are in these positions and push them up high. Have them catch a ball (Fig 3.28) (the 'spider' ball (Fig. A4.32 p. 177) is good for this), hit a ball straight with a rolling pin, play Grip ball or catch toy animals and throw them into a receptacle. Swap each child onto the other piece of equipment after about five minutes (less if one of the children does not like the activity or finds the equipment makes him sore under the arms). A child who can touch the floor can spin herself around on the spot and change direction every 30 seconds. Monitor this input closely, because children can overstimulate themselves with this activity.

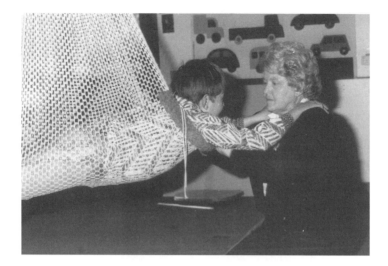

Figure 3.25: 'Flopping down' into a net

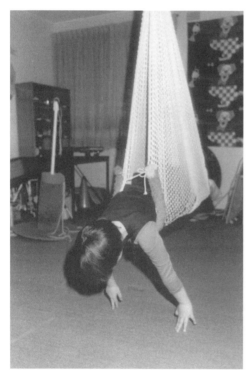

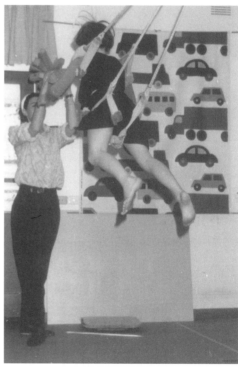

Figure 3.26: A net tied above the child's upper trunk

Figure 3.27: Swinging in a dual swing – 'Superman'

There are two other ways of using the net. One is to have the child hold onto it while she kneels on a scooter board and zooms back and forth (Fig 3.29). The other is to have her hold onto the net and orbit around an inflatable clown or the set of five inner tubes (Fig 3.30).

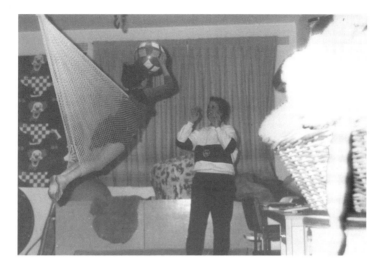

Figure 3.28: Swinging prone in a net and catching a ball

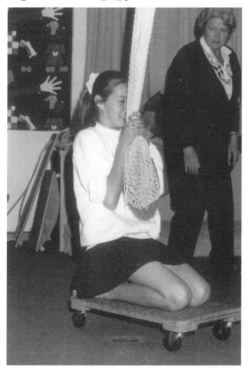

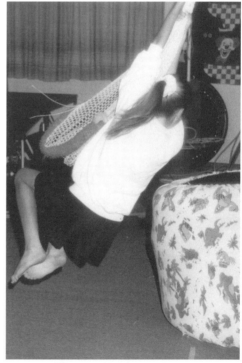

Figure 3.29: Holding a net while zooming on a scooter board

Figure 3.30: Orbiting while holding on to the net

Hitting a suspended ball, sack or small inner tube – bilateral and crossing-the-midline activity

Ask the children to stand either side of a suspended ball, sack or inner tube, holding at each end a rolling pin or a piece of broomstick covered with a variety of textures and taking turns to hit the ball/sack straight to each other (a good bilateral activity). Alternatively, if the children hold the rolling pins at one end, they can take turns to swipe across their body and hit the suspended item. This is a very good crossing-the-midline activity and great fun.

Other bilateral activities are: standing on a balance bubble (or board) and catching a bounced tennis ball between two sink plungers (Fig 3.31); holding a ball between the knees (or ankles) and jumping on spots; holding a ball between the ankles and jumping between straws (Fig 3.32); and playing speedball standing or lying prone (Fig 3.33).

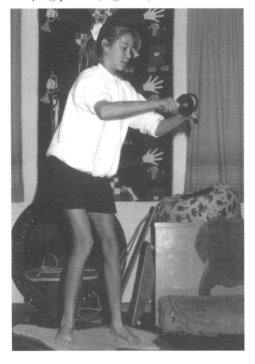

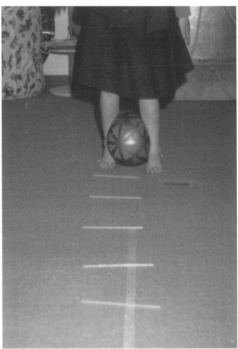

Figure 3.31: Catching a ball with two sink plungers

Figure 3.32: Jumping with a ball between the feet

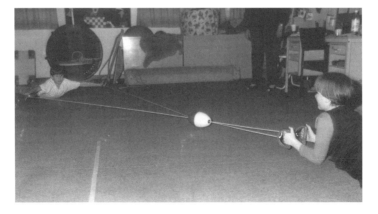

Figure 3.33: Playing speedball while lying prone

Sitting in a net or vertical truck inner tube – rotary movement

Sit one child cross-legged in the net. First, the child straddles the net and puts in one leg (Fig 3.34) and then the other. Spread the net out behind his back and tie the net together with blind cord at each side (Fig 3.35). Sit the other child astride or through the suspended vertical truck inner tube, with her arms around the inner tube itself (Fig 3.36), or ask her to hold on to suspended ropes with handles (Fig 3.37), as she is swung back and forth.

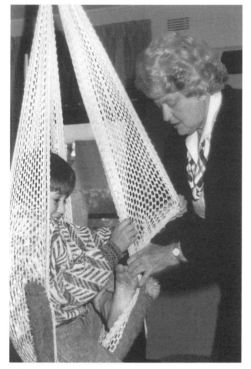

Figure 3.34: Getting into a net, sitting

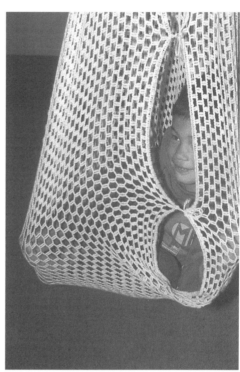

Figure 3.35: A net tied at each side with blind cord

You can also rotate the tube in either an orbit or a spin about its own axis, but ask the child whether she wants orbits, spins or just to go back and forth. Change direction every 30 seconds. Have the child in the net catch small soft toys, accumulate them in the net on his lap and then throw them, one at a time, into a container. He can catch a ball or have a 60 cm inflatable ball thrown at him. Have the child in the inner tube catch the spider ball between her feet (Fig 3.38). After four or five minutes, swap the children's apparatus and activities.

Barrel on a scooter board – balance and eye–hand co-ordination

Have two children stand in a barrel placed on a scooter board. Pull the children around while your assistant throws toy animals, balls and/or beanbags for them to catch, place in the barrel and later throw back into a receptacle.

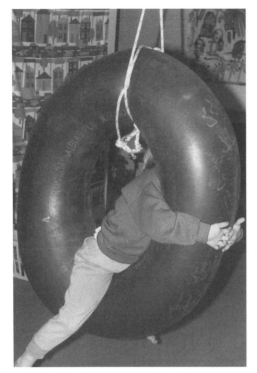

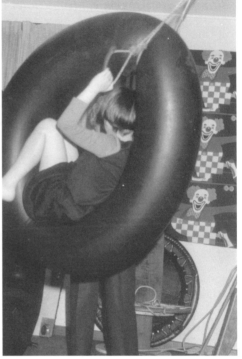

Figure 3.36: Hugging a vertical truck inner tube

Figure 3.37: Swinging in a vertical truck inner tube

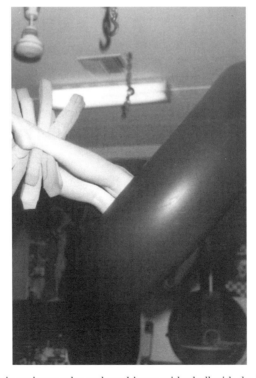

Figure 3.38: Swinging in an inner tube and catching a spider ball with the feet

Inflatable log-bolster – increasing muscle tone and linear movement

Have one child sit or stand (Fig 3.39) at each end of the log bolster and ask the children to bounce up and down alternately. Unless the children can keep themselves on the bolster, an adult should sit behind and bounce with each child. Select ball games such as high toss, throwing a ball around in a circle between children and adults, and rolling balls towards each other on the bolster. A further use of this equipment is for the child to roll along the bolster.

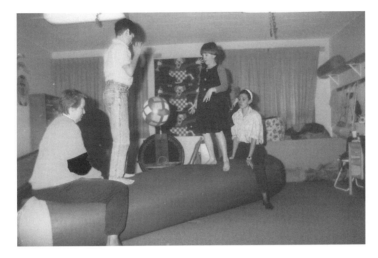

Figure 3.39: Standing on an inflatable log bolster

Bouncing on a mini-trampoline – eye–hand co-ordination, crossing-the-midline and balance

This exercise can be carried out by catching beanbags in a sand bucket, plastic mixing bowl or mini-clothes basket, or by balancing on a curved balance board playing Grip ball and bouncing on the shock-rope 'horse' (Fig 3.40).

Stand the children on the respective equipment and have each one hold the bucket (or a similar container) or Grip ball in each hand. Ask the children to hold their arms apart and then cross them over their bodies. Throw an article (e.g. beanbags into either hand's bucket, or balls onto the Grip ball) while you name the hand. Continue this procedure and call, 'Arms apart' (Fig 3.41), 'Cross your arms over and catch' (Fig 3.42) for about three minutes.

Parachute

The parachute can be used with a group of children (and parents) to achieve elevation of the shoulders (a form of prone extension posture in the upright position). All participants bend down (Fig 3.43) and then bring their arms up above their heads (Fig 3.44). The children can run underneath before the parachute falls down. Young children love this activity.

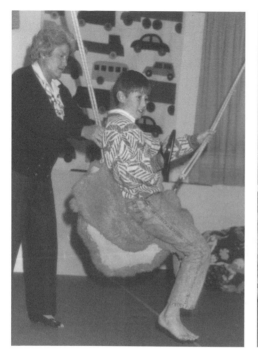

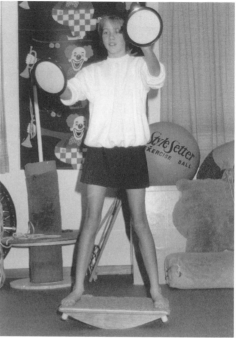

Figure 3.40: Bouncing on a shock-rope horse   **Figure 3.41:** Playing Grip ball – arms apart

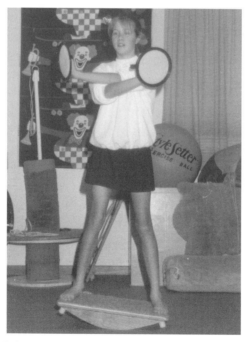

Figure 3.42: Playing Grip ball – arms crossed

Another use of the parachute is to have the children lie across the centre of it and the adults hold the edge of the parachute and move around in a circle, the direction being changed once a full circle has been made.

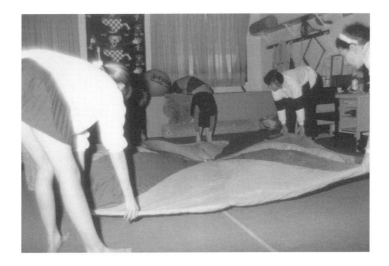

Figure 3.43: Bending down for a game with a parachute

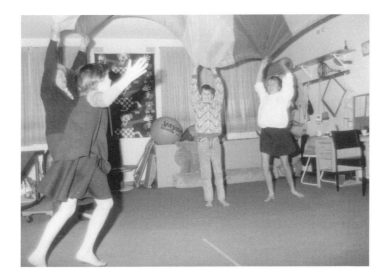

Figure 3.44: Bringing arms up in the air for a game with a parachute

Twister game – protective extension

Occasionally, some children have poor protective extension, usually to the sides, as can be seen during the assessment.

Tell the child to fall onto the named Twister spots. The child learns to fall on her extended arm and thus develops a better protective extension reaction (Fig 3.45).

This 'game' can be fun, especially if two children are involved.

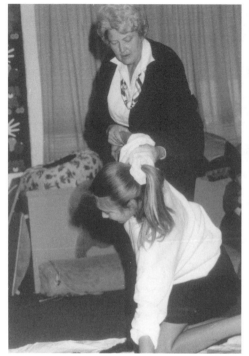

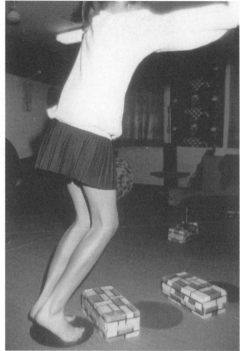

Figure 3.45: Facilitating protective extension on Twister spots

Figure 3.46: Jumping over cardboard bricks onto rubber discs

Gross motor planning

Use some of the many gross motor activities or invent your own, selecting any or all of the following:

- Bounce the ball and jump with the feet together.
- Jump on rubber spots placed between the cardboard bricks (Fig 3.46).
- Jump either side of a rope serpentine path (children can walk along it while crossing their legs or wearing flippers).
- Jump on Twister spots (forward two, back one, forward two, back one and so on). A similar mat made of cotton with spots of different textures makes the activity more tactually stimulating. This mat needs to be used on carpet to keep it stable.
- Jump with an animal or a balloon between the ankles and zig zag either side of a line on the floor.
- Jump with a soft ball between the ankles in a figure-of-eight design around 'witches' hats' (Fig 3.47).
- Move around the room pretending to be an animal such as a rabbit, duck, crab, frog, bucking donkey or kangaroo.
- Pretend to be a pirate with only one eye and one leg.
- Lie on a carpet and form numbers or letters with body.
- Play 'Simon says'.
- With the feet together, jump in and out of cane hoops forwards, sideways and backwards.

- Walk in unusual patterns, for example using the knee of one leg and the foot of another, having the knees slightly bent or walking like a toy soldier, with the same arm and leg moving together (not reciprocally, as is the normal walking pattern).
- Jump back and forth over a slowly moving rope (like a snake).
- Place a long rope on the floor, the rope often crossing over itself. Walk along the rope, jumping over each crossing.
- Have the child on his hands and knees on the scooter board, one arm and one leg off the scooter board pushing on the floor, and one arm and one leg on the scooter board (Fig 3.48). This activity can be included with ramp work, when returning to the top of the ramp after zooming down.

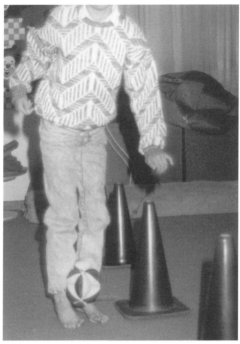

Figure 3.47: Jumping in a figure-of-eight around 'witches' hats

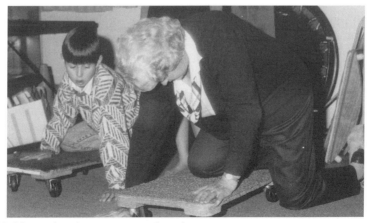

Figure 3.48: Motor planning on a scooter board

- Jump along a line on a space hopper (Fig 3.49).
- Walk on a cable roller on its side, upgrading this to simultaneously catching and bouncing a ball (Fig 3.50).

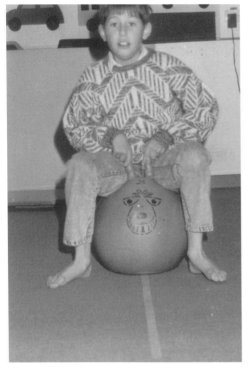 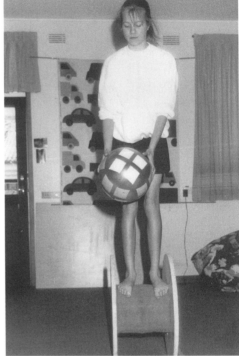

Figure 3.49: Jumping on a space hopper   **Figure 3.50:** Walking on a cable roller

Gross visual space perception

Select any or all of the following activities to create an obstacle course (Fig 3.51):

- Crawling through cane or plastic hoops, car inner tubes or a plastic tunnel.
- Crawling around chairs in a figure-of-eight pattern, the children first seeing where they are going and later having a paper bag over their heads to occlude their vision.
- Crawling under and over the ramp.
- Lying on the scooter boards and propelling themselves between the legs of tables or chairs – backwards, forwards, prone and supine.
- Crawling around obstacle boxes.
- Crawling under the raised mini-trampoline, which has six legs, one pair of opposite legs being folded up and the other four legs raised on cardboard bricks (Fig 3.51).
- Including motor planning activities and/or visual space perception games that have motor planning components, because motor planning and visual space perception interrelate.

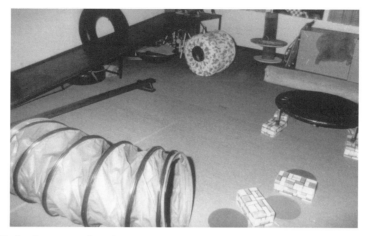

Figure 3.51: Setting up an obstacle course

Fine motor/visual space skills

Fine motor skills should be carried out while the child is moving gently because these activities provide multisensory input for more effective integration. The child sits on the bolster swing, inflatable log bolster or tractor inner tube, and you sit on it with him and move the equipment.

Activities can be selected from the following:

- Cut out or create different shapes from coloured play-dough.
- Use Theraplast, Blu-Tack or play-dough to make a long 'snake' and roll it into a snail (Fig 3.52). With Exercise putty, make the outline of a face, the eyes, eyebrows, mouth and nose.
- Match hand shapes on cards using a selection of bright yellow cards on which you have drawn a variety of black hand shapes. The hands can be curled hands or have one or two fingers or the thumb abducted – any variety of hand postures will do. The child has to place his hands on the cards in these abnormal positions.
- Thread beads – any sized beads, macaroni, plastic tubing cut into small pieces, buttons, bottle tops or thin strips of coloured paper rolled around a knitting needle – to make a necklace.
- Create mosaics.
- Play the game 'boxes' or follow a maze on the white/blackboard.
- Sew around designs on cards (using old greeting cards).
- Play commercially available fine motor games, such as Lego, Duplo, Meccano, peg-in-the-hole games, interlocking building blocks and constructional games.
- Weave paper strips or make paper chains.
- Make collages from strips torn out of magazines, shells, leaves, macaroni, string and coloured wool.
- Play dot-to-dot and line games.
- Make articles from matchsticks or lolly sticks.

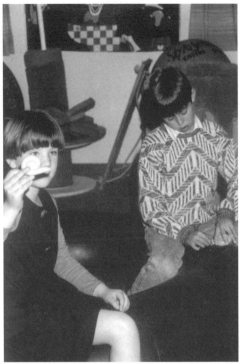

Figure 3.52: Making a snail out of Exercise putty

Fine visual space perception activities

Select from the following:

- Match picture cards or numbers and pictures on overturned playing cards ('memories').
- Play 'Chinese Checkers' whereby the child copies a design by moving little coloured balls into the holes.
- Copy or create designs on geoboard (a board with round-headed nails inserted into the board 25 cm apart, both vertically and horizontally) with rubber bands.
- Copy a design that you have constructed from coloured blocks; varying the complexity.
- Construct designs with wooden geometric shapes.
- Copy letters, numbers or a design in wet sand or shaving foam.

Calming

Calm all children at the conclusion of the session so that they leave feeling relaxed and manageable (for their parents or teachers). Some children need to be calmed because they are very active; if this is the case, introduce fine motor and fine visual space activities, which are all-absorbing, prior to or with the calming activities.

Select from the following calming techniques:

- Slow movement and deep pressure – hold the younger child in your lap and gently rock him while he watches something intriguing (a sand window, bubble novelties, egg timers, preferably with different lengths of time). He may resist sitting in your lap if he is tactually defensive. If so, put him in a rocking chair.

- Sit him or lie him along the bolster swing and slowly rock the bolster back and forth, or place him across the bolster with his head lowered. Stroke down either side of his vertebral column with your index and middle fingers (Fig 3.53, 3.54 and 3.55), vibrate over his back (Fig 3.56) or stroke him with your hands or tactile objects (a brush, piece of sheepskin, feather duster or paint brush). Alternatively, place a large toy animal or roll a 30 cm inflatable ball on top of the child while he is lying prone (especially if the child does not like human contact); at the same time, move him gently back and forth on the bolster.

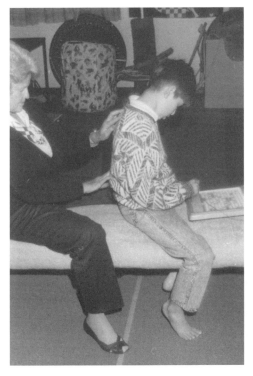 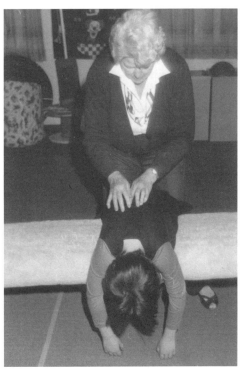

Figure 3.53: Being stroked while sitting and moving

Figure 3.54: Being stroked while in an inverted position

- Lie him on a sheepskin on the floor and roll a large therapy ball (at least 90 cm in diameter) firmly over him (Fig 3.57). Lean quite heavily on the ball as you roll it.
- Lie the child in a large net and swing her slowly and gently back and forth and round.
- Sit her in a net and hold her firmly while you move her gently back and forth and round (Fig 3.58).
- Sit the child in a slightly deflated large therapy ball and move the ball gently in all directions (Fig 3.59).
- Lie the child on a sheepskin in the Gigantos saucer and gently move the saucer.
- Sit the child in a rocking chair and slowly rock it.

- Lying in a large box of durable plastic balls (see Fig 3.1 p. 37) can be very rest-ful for some children.

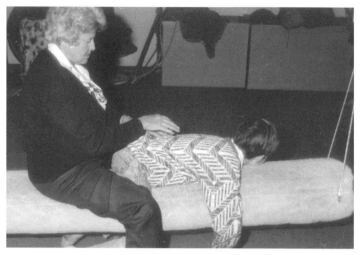

Figure 3.55: Stroking down either side of the vertebral column

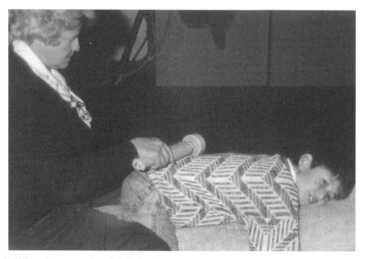

Figure 3.56: Vibrating over the child's back to calm him

Remember that the activity should be pleasant and relaxing for the child or it may elicit a tactually defensive response.

Ending the session

At the conclusion of the treatment session, after the child has put on his socks and shoes, and if he deserves it, offer a choice of stickers or a stamp on the hand. Most young children look forward to this reward. Offer older children a merit award card with an appropriate message and sticker on it.

Lack of progress

If a child is not progressing and there is no apparent reason for this, you may need to go back a step and provide lower-level activities. Select simple tactile, vestibular-

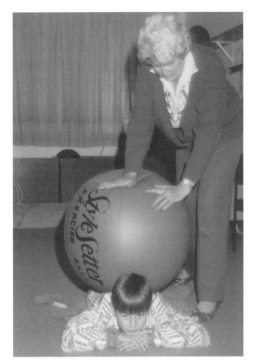

Figure 3.57: Having deep pressure from a ball to calm a child

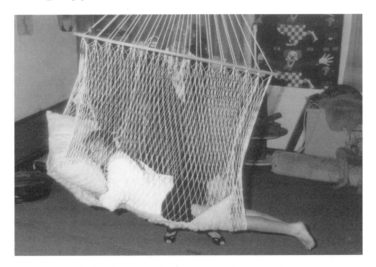

Figure 3.58: Rocking gently in a large net hammock to calm a child

proprioceptive activities that also provide simple visual and auditory stimulation. Alternatively, the child may need a break: some children benefit from four-to-six week break from therapy midway through the block. After such a break, the child's nervous system is usually ready to respond again.

Not all children and families are helped by occupational therapy, but explore all avenues and then make appropriate referrals. A significant contribution from an occupational therapist is to decide when a child or family needs other professional help and to refer them to the appropriate specialist(s).

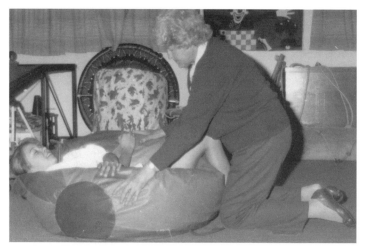

Figure 3.59: Lying in a deflated ball and rocking to calm a child

Managing specific deficits

Despite appropriate and careful monitoring you may on occasions encounter some of the following deficits among children whom you treat:

* low tolerance to movement
* nausea
* headache
* high tolerance to movement
* tactile defensiveness
* intolerance of noise, light or smell
* bedwetting
* overactivity, distractibility, poor concentration, irritability or fussiness
* gravitational insecurity
* speech deficits.

Low tolerance to movement

This can be observed in the Southern California Postrotary Nystagmus Test or in the treatment session (Fisher *et al.*, 1991). Monitor vestibular-proprioceptive stimulation, even self-activating stimulation. Say 'Stop' or observe them closely and intervene. The effects of vestibular–proprioceptive stimulation (nausea, vomiting, headaches and other autonomic nervous system signs) can be delayed. Overstimulation can induce seizures.

If the child's tolerance to movement is low, avoid giving her specific vestibular activities, especially those involving rotary movements. Use other sensory channels and give her activities that have a tactile/proprioceptive basis, such as applying pressure on the shoulders while she is on the balance board. Have her hit a ball or walk around a tractor inner tube, or roll a large therapy ball over her and apply firm pressure.

Many children with low vestibular tolerance can tolerate linear activities. Try the child on the ramp, or try lying or sitting her on the bolster swing while applying pressure to her back; alternatively, have her jump on the mini-trampoline and catch toy animals. As soon as the child mentions discomfort or shows signs of not tolerating the movement, stop the activity immediately.

Concentrate on activities that involve eye–hand co-ordination because the visual system can contribute to neural inhibition. The child's tolerance to movement rarely improves with treatment but, by carefully selecting activities, you can work round the problem. Watch for signs such as pallor, sweating and sudden quietness. Warn the child about sometimes feeling sick and ask him to tell you straight away so that you can stop. Be particularly aware of the child with a strong need to please. Often he will not say he is feeling unwell because he 'badly' wants to complete or achieve what you have asked. If you see the signs, step in and change immediately to a calming activity.

Nausea

Nausea can be stopped in the following ways:

*   Massage the base of the occiput just above the nuchal ligaments (Fig 3.60).
*   Play a game of push o'war (as opposed to tug o'war) in which the child and a sibling, friend or parent go onto their hands and knees and, in this position, push on a ball or pillow placed between the tops of their heads (Fig 3.61).

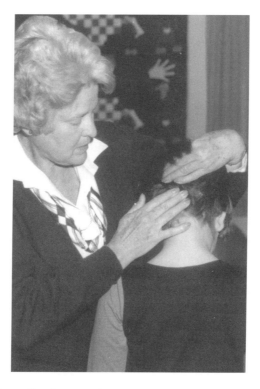

Figure 3.60: Massaging base of occiput to reduce nausea

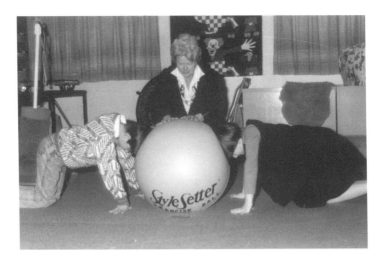

Figure 3.61: Pressing heads against a ball to reduce nausea

- Fixate on an object, for example, the moving minute hand of a watch or catch and throw a ball, the ball going in all directions.
- Breathe deeply.
- Press above the child's upper lip with an index finger placed parallel to the lips for six seconds on the lip (Fig 3.62) and six seconds off the lip. Continue to repeat this until the symptoms have subsided.

Headache

Control treatment-related headache in one of the following ways:

- Apply pressure above the child's upper lip (as described for nausea).
- Advise the child to shower or swim in cold water if the headache is still present when he gets home.
- Suggest that the child avoids any bouncing activities.
- Modify further treatment sessions to avoid recurrence of these effects.

High tolerance to movement

Some children have high tolerance to movement and can spin endlessly. High tolerance to movement indicates poor sensory processing and, unless this processing can be improved, treatment will be ineffective. If the child's vision is occluded, activities that involve tactile, vestibular–proprioceptive input improve integration; this improvement seems to make the child's tolerance to movement more normal.

To treat a child with high vestibular tolerance, fit an eye shade or tie a scarf around the eyes while he carries out rotary (vestibular–proprioceptive) activities (Fig 3.63). Remove the eye shade or scarf if the child suddenly feels nauseous. Recommend self-activating and home programme activities such as spinning in a net, spinning on a horizontal car tyre or spinning himself in a truck inner tube vertically suspended.

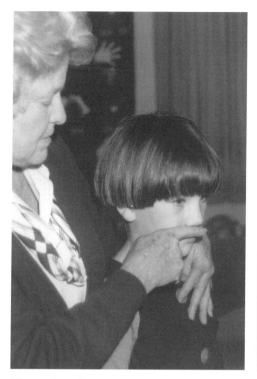

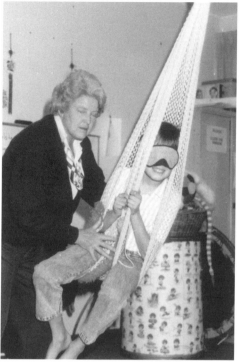

Figure 3.62: Pressing on the upper lip to reduce nausea or headache

Figure 3.63: Using a blindfold to reduce high tolerance to movement

Tactile defensiveness

A child is tactually defensive if she has the tendency to respond negatively or aversively to certain types of tactile stimulus (Royeen and Lane, 1991, p. 108). Current thinking suggests that this is one form of sensory defensiveness.

A tactually defensive child finds activities involving light touch very uncomfortable; she may avoid even loving touch, overreact to being bumped or brushed against, feel uncomfortable at the closeness of others if standing in a queue, fear or dislike certain people or house pets, avoid acts such as hair cuts, hairwashing, bathing or being barefoot or messy, and avoid some kinds of clothing, toys or textures (especially soft ones) (Price, 1978, Royeen and Lane, 1991). Tactile stimulation can be painful for children with low tactile threshold. Do not give them tactile activities they do not like.

When a tactually defensive child finds such sensations unpleasant, his response is primal. He will pull his hand away from yours or occasionally hit back at you if you are too close as you work with him. The responses may be immediate, automatic and unpremeditated – often exaggerated – physical withdrawal, or resistance and hitting back. He may also make a civilised comment such as 'I want to go now' as an indication of discomfort (Price, 1978).

Use the other sensory channels and provide vestibular–proprioceptive activities with deep pressure. Have the child cling to the flexor swing and catch toys, or swing in the net hammock. Provide compression to the lower limb joints through the child's extended legs while she lies prone in the net or dual swing. Have her jump up and down on the tractor inner tube and catch beanbags in a bucket. Also use activities that involve visual and auditory senses. Encourage the child to select and initiate tactile activities (Sears, 1981).

Avoid exposing the child to unpleasant tactile stimulation. Exposure does not increase tolerance but rather stimulates adrenaline release and worsens the reaction. Explanations are usually ineffective because the child's reaction is a primal, survival reaction. Attempts at behaviour modification are usually also ineffective. Try firm rhythmic rubbing to decrease the sensitivity, but warn the child that a touch is coming. Slowly rock and roll the child (because any smooth movement helps to lower resistance). Use firm pressure, rather than soft touch, while holding him.

The child can sometimes overheat. If this occurs, cool the child with cold water or place ice in her mouth. Suggest that parents allow the child to chose her hairstyle, clothing (wearing more or less than the current season normally requires), bathing methods, pets and toys (Price, 1978). Explain to the family that the phenomenon is a reaction of the nervous system that the child cannot control, but be aware that mothers may feel guilty when their babies or children reject them physically. Punishing the child will not help; a calm response is important.

Some information about tactile defensiveness for teachers is worthwhile, especially about warning the child when they will be touching him and in case the child displays tactually defensive reactions in school, for example hitting back at another child should he get too close. Teachers can also assist the child to adjust to the school environment by allowing him to stand at the end of lines and sit at the back of the class. Additionally, the child will be comfortable if he is approached front-on and at eye level (Sears, 1981).

Note that, if the child is tactually defensive, no amount of 'conditioning' will lessen that adrenaline-charged tactually defensive reaction. Deep touch and pressure contacts adapt more readily than other forms of touch, so the tactfully defensive child may respond more readily to deep touch. Try pressing a large cushion on her or rolling a large ball over her.

Intolerance of noise, light or smell

Children who do not tolerate noise, light or smell may be disinhibited and unable to suppress responses to these stimuli. Select activities that avoid the unpleasant stimulus until the disinhibition lessens.

Bedwetting

Most children achieve bladder control by the age of four years. Children who continue to wet the bed beyond this age may be helped by the following interventions. Ensure that the child is calm prior to going to bed in order to get the parasympathetic system operating (Rood, personal communication, 1976).

If necessary, use the calming techniques described above. Place a beach towel, large toy or 'bolster' alongside the child. A bolster can be made by wrapping two pillows in a beach towel. Pin the towel first to check whether it is successful and then sew it. Restrict the child's late-evening drinking. Eliminate all milk products and concentrated fruit juice from the child's diet for two weeks. Some children are sensitive to these foods, and this sensitivity can contribute to their bedwetting. Children are occasionally sensitive to chemicals in water, so it is not necessarily the amount of water consumed that is causing the problem. The family may be able to purchase a water purifier if they are suspicious of chemicals in their water.

Overactivity, distractibility, poor concentration, fussiness and irritability

These behaviours of disinhibition usually lessen as treatment progresses and the inhibitory areas of the nervous system become more efficient. Occasionally, however, a sensitivity to food(s), chemical(s) or water is the underlying cause (see Chapter 5).

Overactivity

A general stimulation programme should improve inhibition and lessen overactivity. However, it is important for the child to be calmed for about 10 minutes at the end of the treatment session.

Calm the child with slow rocking and deep pressure techniques as used at the end of a treatment session (see above).

Distractibility and poor concentration

If the child is tired through having late nights or poor sleep patterns, he will have poor concentration. Food or chemical sensitivities (see Chapter 5) have the same effect. Whatever the cause, a child who is easily distractible or who has poor concentration will have even more difficulty in learning.

For distractibility and poor concentration at school, ask the teacher to seat the child at the front of the class to avoid distraction from his classmates. It is essential that he is comfortable at his desk and that the chair is the correct height, his feet being firmly on the floor. A sheepskin on the seat can add tactile awareness. If these items of furniture are not suitable, the child will not be posturally stable and will fidget. Proximal stability is basic to the fine motor skills required for schoolwork; if not attended to, this will result in his not being able to concentrate properly. French (personal communication, 1993) suggests that the teacher mark an area with masking tape on the floor for the child's boundaries when he is sitting on the floor. For homework, have him in a quiet room free of distractors such as radio, television, other members of the family and toys. McFadden (1988) suggests introducing practice for concentration by challenging the child to complete a certain amount of work within a set time (measured by a kitchen timer), increasing the period of required concentration as he progresses. Give him positive reinforcement and a reward if he achieves this. Use the same 'contract' principles as mentioned on p. 36.

To help the child concentrate on his homework, suggest to the parents that the child does some home programme activities (see Appendix 3). Follow this stimulation with a homework period. It is advisable for you to discuss with the class teacher what is a realistic amount of time to spend on homework, particularly if it turns into a battle between parents and the child (French, personal communication, 1993).

The importance for the child to have a routine needs to be emphasised. This will help to settle him and concentrate both at home and at school (French, personal communication, 1993).

Irritability and fussiness

There is no specific treatment for irritability and fussiness if these are caused by disinhibition alone. They usually decrease with the treatment applied for major deficit(s).

Gravitational insecurity

Let the child be in control and do the activity herself. Provide activities in which her feet can touch the floor, if she wants, such as sitting on a low bolster swing, lying across a truck inner tube, running back and forth catching a ball, being on a flexor swing that is very low to the ground or being on equipment that is actually on the floor, such as the Sit'n'spin (Fig 3.64) or five inner tubes barrel. Never force the child onto high equipment if she shows fear or protests. Gravitational insecurity lessens dramatically after a period of therapy, and this change indicates that therapy is having an overall beneficial effect.

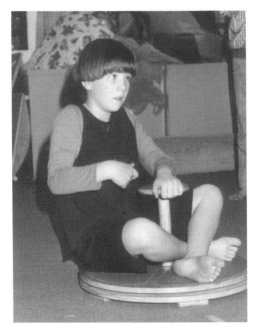

Figure 3.64: Sitting on a Sit'n'spin for gravitational insecurity

Speech deficits

Combined occupational therapy and speech therapy sessions have been most successful for children who have marked speech problems and learning and/or co-ordination difficulties. Give older children (6 to 9 years) faster occupational therapy activities with multisensory input without speech therapy. Do this for the first third of the session. For the remainder of the session, give slow, gentle activities such as moving on the bolster swing, inflatable log bolster, horizontal tyre or tractor inner tube, while the child is undergoing speech therapy. Give younger children (3–6 years) short sessions (of approximately 10 minutes) of faster activities in occupational therapy, then again slow activities with speech therapy. Repeat the procedure with smaller children. This allows for a break from the cortical concentration needed during speech therapy.

Combined therapy with multisensory input is much more effective as a basis for speech therapy than having children sitting still. Speech therapists who have combined their treatment in this way report very favourably on their clients' outcomes.

Low self-esteem

Children who are having problems with learning and co-ordination usually have low self-esteem, so this is an important area of treatment to which parents should be alerted. The Coopersmith assessment (see Chapter 2, p. 24) provides a good evaluation a few weeks after therapy sessions have commenced. By this stage, the children have learned to trust you and the parents respect you sufficiently to listen to your advice, especially if you have some definite Coopersmith test results to show them. This assessment is able to identify more clearly in which environment the child's self-esteem is low – in school, at home or in general.

Encourage people to speak to the child in a positive way, for example. 'You did quite well in your test this week. Next week, let's see whether you can get one more word right' (French, personal communication, 1993). Provide *sincere* praise and positive feedback. Children are acutely aware of body language and usually sense and respond to that more than to words. French also found that these children often did not know how to accept positive feedback. Thus, in the treatment session, she often practised, via role-play or an activity, the giving and receiving of praise. For example, have one child jump on the mini-trampoline and everyone else stands around him. Each person in the room (including therapist and parents) takes it in turn to jump on the mini-trampoline. Throw a ball to the jumping person and give him a compliment, such as, 'I like your blue shirt.' He then throws the ball back and has to return a compliment. It is important to include the parents in this because they are often not good at being positive towards their children.

French (personal communication, 1993) recommends encouraging parents and teachers to identify something that their children are good at and follow through those skills as hobbies. Children need this balance, particularly because their schoolwork is so poor and they have failed so often.

Parents and their children need to sit down and work out a list of responsibilities for home tasks, which help to make the children feel worthwhile contributors to family life. If the children are older, the parents can formulate a written contract between them and the children, which makes it seem even more important.

If parents do not reinforce good self-esteem, all the reinforcement from others is far less effective. First and foremost, children want their *parents* to think they are great.

Children with poor social skills need to develop verbal and eye contact with both the teacher and other people. Start by role-play with the mother and father, and then with siblings, family or close friends. The mother may then get the teacher similarly to practise verbal and eye contact.

Teasing

Children who 'fail' are teased: by their peers, in the playground, on the bus, on their way to and from school or by their siblings. Sibling teasing is common in most families and is healthy, but children with problems are more affected by this and need to be able to handle it, being one extra thing they have to contend with. No-one likes to be teased (hurtfully), whether one is 8 or 58. Teasers are often bullies, attention-seekers or ring leaders who are trying to detract from their own inadequacies. It is helpful to find out who are the main teasers and counsel the child as to why these children may be acting this way. Suggest to parents that they obtain the support of the child's teacher.

It is advisable to point out to the child that *anyone* can be teased about *anything* – having red hair; wearing glasses; being overweight, tall, short or skinny; coming from an ethnic background; talking 'posh' – the list is endless. How the teased person *deals* with the teasing is the crucial factor. If he acts upset or hurt, the teasing will continue; if he is off-hand and not worried, or makes a joke of it, everyone becomes bored by the exercise, the teasing loses its effect and it therefore ceases.

Teasing and low self-esteem usually go together. If the child's self-esteem can be improved, she is likely to cope better with teasing, both at home and at school. Therefore encourage parents and family to build the child's self-esteem. However, as seen in Chapter 4, every family member is affected in some way by the child with the problem, and siblings frequently tease the problem child (who has had more attention from the parents) simply because they too are endeavouring to gain their share of their parents' attention. This becomes a vicious circle. One other suggestion for home is to have the parents write a list of the good *character* points (rather than 'She has pretty curly hair') of *every child in the family*, not just the child with the problem. Suggest that the parents put these lists on the fridge and every day tell those children – *sincerely* – about their good points and good character traits. The parents will probably feel better about their children and keep unimportant issues, such as clothes being left on the floor, in proportion. With improvement in the children's self-esteem, interaction is more positive and they can handle the teasing better. Thus a 'laid-back' attitude can be seen. If appropriate, and if the family is a 'team', suggest that Mum and Dad have a list too – made by the children (and prompted by their parents if necessary). This encourages the children to think about their parents' qualities.

Another successful strategy has been to role-play, impromptu, without warning, both in the treatment sessions and at home. Get the children to practise saying, and *sincerely* meaning, the inoffensive reply 'So what?' The teaser says, 'You run funny.' The child replies (off-hand), 'So what?' It is important for the teased child to get the message over to the teasers that he really does not care. Intensive role-play can be very effective. The child has to feel 'OK' with his parents so that he does not get hurt by *their* role-play 'teasing'.

Should the child be teased by a group in the playground, in the bus or walking home from school, he is advised to play close to the supervising teacher on playground duty, to sit near the bus driver or to walk home with friends. It may be necessary for him to be taken or collected by car until he is more able to handle the teasing.

The last resort is changing schools, but this may make a great deal of difference to the child's school and emotional progress; he starts afresh with a new set of friends and teachers.

Group sessions, held weekly, have been very successful in helping children to improve their self-esteem and deal with teasing. Group camps, held for one week each year, have also been most beneficial.

Treating children with other disabilities

A sensory integrative approach to treatment can be applied to children with other types of dysfunction and (in a modified form) to adults with an intellectual disability or emotional disturbance. If you work with children or adults in these categories, modify their programme to meet their different needs. The resultant programme is in the form of sensory stimulation whereby different areas of the brain may be stimulated and the therapy given for different reasons, but the therapeutic procedures are very similar. These principles can be applied by therapists working outside the learning disability field with highly beneficial results.

When you treat a child with increased tone, place him in a posture opposite to that of his hypertonic posture. For example, if a child has high extensor tone, have him sit in a large box, in a flexed position and go down the ramp, but do not have him go down the ramp in the prone position. If the hypertonus affects the trunk and limb flexors, employ prone extension activities that involve the scooter board, the large therapy ball, the net and/or the dual swing. Any temporary increase in tone will be quickly reversed once the activity ceases, and these types of stimulation yield numerous sustained benefits. After each treatment session, seek feedback from the parents of these children about any after-effects, both positive and negative.

Conclusion

The above programmes are only **suggestions** for treatment and overall management. Many excellent books have been written on the subject; reading these can add appropriate information to your experience. You are also advised to seek appropriate training in sensory integration theory and practice.

Such children are a sheer delight to treat. Their families are an inspiration, and you will find that the children and their parents will be some of your best teachers. It is one of the most exciting and rewarding fields of work. The joy is boundless.

References and recommended reading

Ayres A J (1979) *Sensory Integration and the Child*. Los Angeles: Western Psychological Services.

Biddulph S (1988) *The Secret of Happy Children*. Kensington, Sydney: Bay Books.

Canter L, Canter M (1988) *Assertive Discipline for Parents*. New York: Harper & Row. Now out of print, but obtainable from Denise Nicholls, Behaviour Management Australia, Unit 37, Como Corporate Centre, Cnr Mary and Preston Sts. Como, WA 6152.

Cocks N (1992) *Skipping Not Tripping*. Sydney: Simon Schuster.

Dobson J (1983) *Discipline While You Can*. Eastbourne: Kingsway Publications.

Dreikurs R (1982) *Happy Children – A Challenge to Parents*. London: Souvenir Press.

Fisher AG, Murray EA, Bundy AC (1991) *Sensory Integration: Theory and Practice*. Philadelphia: Davis p. 102.

Green C (1985) *Toddler Taming: A Parents' Guide to (Surviving) the First Few Years*. Sydney: Macarthur Press.

Jordan DR (1988) *Attention Deficit Disorder – ADD Syndrome*. Austin: Pro-Ed.

McFadden J (1988) *The Simple Way to Raise a Good Kid*. Sydney: Martin Educational.

Martin G, Pear J (1988) *Behaviour Modification. What It Is and How To Do It*. Englewood Cliffs, NJ: Prentice Hall.

Price AJ (1978) Tactile defensiveness: hypersensitivity to touch. *International Study Group for Perception Bulletin* 3:1.

Royeen CB, Lane SJ (1991) Tactile processing and sensory defensiveness. In Fisher AG, Murray EA, Bundy AC (eds). *Sensory Integration: Theory and Practice*. Philadelphia: Davis. pp. 108–21.

Sears C (1981) The tactile defensive child. *Academic Therapy* 16: 563–9.

Sellers JS (1989) *Motor Development Program for School-Age Children*. Tuscon: Therapy Skill Builders.

Serfontein G (1992) *The Hidden Handicap. How to Help Children who Suffer from Dyslexia, Hyperactivity and Learning Difficulties*. Sydney: Simon Schuster.

Tickle-Degman AG, Coster W (1995) Therapeutic interaction and the management of challenge during the beginning minutes of sensory integration treatment. *Occupational Therapy Journal of Research* 15:2, 122.

Chapter 4
Behaviour Management in Young Children: A Therapist's Guide for Parents

Joanna Nicklin

Handling other people's children is often a lot easier than handling our own, because we are not so emotionally attached; we can stand back, and we see the whole family situation dispassionately. To a non-involved adult, it is obvious why each person behaves in the way he or she does.

Meeting with parents

In some families, handling is ineffective, and ineffectiveness usually causes unhappiness that can easily affect all the relationships. Therapists have something to offer these families: they can help to 'tidy up behaviour'.

Begin by developing an effective relationship with the client. When I first meet a family, I explain to them what we hope to achieve in the therapy to be administered and how I propose to go about handling the behaviour of the child so that I can achieve the required aims. If I sense anxiety in the parents, I need to isolate the specific areas that worry them, be these in therapy and the way it is administered or in the way in which I propose to control the situation. I may have to arrange for the parents to come alone to a special session to explain the 'tools of management', so that they will totally support my efforts when treatment starts.

Parents must not bring along even a suckling baby, because any distractions reduce the amount they gain from this session, they simply cannot concentrate when their offspring are opening drawers, talking or even quietly playing. Arrange interim babysitting, out of hearing range or ask the parents to arrange for a babysitter. If they make this commitment, they will really come, ready to learn. I have found that if I allow even the smallest infringement, the session is less effective.

Tape the session and give the parents the tape at the end so that they can replay it later if they start to revert to their old ways. One takes in only 20% of new material at the first session, so the tape will help with recall. Mothers have told me that the tape helps greatly. I also give the parents a diagram (Table 4.1) to stick on their refrigerator, to remind them, often mid-fight, how to rectify the problem.

Table 4.1: Tools of management

Anticipate
    Basic needs
    Routine

Handle conflict
    Respond in the beginning
    Withdraw
    Use body language
    Be dramatic
    Carry the child

Repair the damage
    Intervene and distract
    Take responsibility for our actions
    Try again
    Earn the right

Be consistent
    Parents do their best, but best varies every day
    Allow children to make mistakes
    Let children grow emotionally

It is vitally important, wherever possible, to see both parents together. For a one-parent family, include the support people – grandparents, partners, anybody to whom the single parent can turn for help. These people whether they are at the initial interview or not, must not undermine the parents' efforts to succeed. If there is no support, treatment is unlikely to be successful because the child then has two bosses. The child can 'play' one off against the other and the relationship will be damaged.

Family dynamics

If you are a therapist skilled in working with families, you may wish to use the following procedures. However, inexperienced therapists are **strongly cautioned** that a mishandled situation can cause distress.

Start the session by talking about family dynamics because clients need to understand how important it is to have all the caring people at the interview. No-one should feel that he or she is being 'talked about' or 'run down'. Each person should be ready to be part of the team.

Draw a circle and say, 'This is Dad', or Mum, or whoever is sitting there in front of you. Draw all the authority figures and then draw in the children. We are going to consider a traditional household where there is a child with a problem.

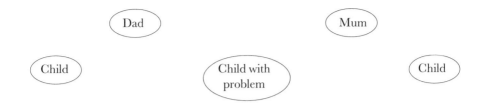

If I sense that the family is too threatened to be represented on paper, I create a family with several children and a problem – deafness, blindness or poor behaviour. The real problem child may just be a spoilt younger child, an only boy or an only girl, and it is much better if they can accept their own family diagram.

The next step is to draw lines between the circles. Beside the problem child, draw a little black circle and say, 'This child has a few problems. This is the child who has been pretty hard to live with, so the whole family has had to make adjustments. These adjustments are not always the best for the family or the child, but they have just happened for the sake of survival.' Then fill in the little black circle beside the 'problem' child. Continue by saying, 'So a lot of attention, be it good or bad, goes to this child.' At the same time, draw lines, leading from each adult to this child. This extra attention can build up a lot of resentment among the other children. No-one needs to take the blame for this extra attention, because survival is the name of the game, but it is very destructive to any other children and their relationships with parents and that child. If left unchecked, these other children can grow up very resentful of this child and often leave home very young and ill-prepared. They leave to escape the chaos. Draw a little black circle beside each other child saying, 'Each child has an extra little problem, because he or she has to put up with this child in the family.'

Give the family time to look at this diagram, and then draw lines from the adult to the other children, saying, 'So we have to make sure that these children get the same amount and quality of attention as this first one.'

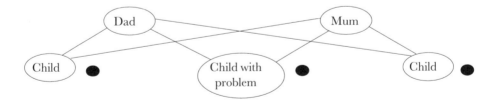

Continue by drawing another little black circle beside Dad (or the male head of the household): say, 'So Dad has one, equally as big, because he worries about his little family.' He goes out and tries to provide, but he goes out! He is not with the children all the time, so that when he comes back, he might be tired but he can look at how the family is functioning as something of an outsider and can often see, much more clearly than Mum, what is happening. Warn Dads that this is **not** the time to tell Mum that she's not doing it correctly but to pitch in and help her. There will be time to give advice later!

Look at the Mum and say, 'Draw a huge black circle. The Mums have one too, but theirs is huge. It sometimes threatens to engulf them totally.'

Mothers will often cry at this point, so keep a box of tissues handy. Don't stop, but gently and quietly push the tissues into the mother's reach and continue: 'They don't get out, they are on duty 24 hours a day. Sure, they sometimes go overboard, or are too soft, but they have no choice, they are stuck with the problem non-stop, so let's look at Mum.' With a pencil poised say, pointing to Mum's big black circle, 'Who is the most important person in this family? Not this child' and point to the problem one, 'or these children, or even Dad, although he has his worries. It's Mum.' Draw a box around Mum and say, 'What happens to this family if anything happens to Mum? We have to look after her.' Look at the spouse/partner and say, 'You married her' or 'You're with her because you love her,' drawing a line across from Mum to Dad. Continue to draw lines between the two, making quite a thick rope of lines and saying, 'You're married (or together), because you loved each other; let's hope that feeling is still as strong when all these are gone' (drawing a long line separating the parents from all the children). 'Let's hope this relationship is as strong, or stronger after they are gone, as it was before they came. Work on it. Make time for it. It might mean time just talking together, but be careful not to neglect this relationship. You are still the same lovely people underneath, after all these years. Let me help you get the handling of the children tidied up.' No parents want unruly, unpleasant children. They would prefer to have nice ones if they could; they just don't know how.

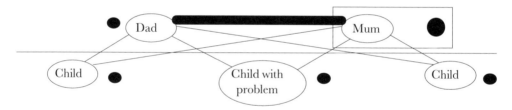

Tools of management

Say to the parents, 'I can't tell you how to bring up your children, I have no right to do that, but I can offer you the "tools of management", so that you can put it together for yourselves within your own family structure.' Give the parents the sheet of the four guidelines (Table 4.1) and explain the steps.

There are seven key steps towards helping a family handle their children:

- **anticipate**
- **handle conflict**
  - manage behaviour
  - withdraw
- **repair the damage**
  - earn the right
- **be consistent.**

The last step, *being consistent*, is the hardest. It seems straightforward but, because we were 'imprinted' by our own parents and their own handling of us, we slip back into our familiar behaviour patterns when we are pushed to the brink by our children. Although we think thoughts such as, 'I'll never do that to my children,' we often do just that, because we work on 'automatic pilot' so much of the time. We can change, but it takes time. Both parents need to work with each other, but be gentle with their feelings and pride; offer parents a face-saving way out.

Anticipate

Basic needs

Understand and recognise that a child has *basic needs* for sleep, food and feeling needed. If you fight with a tired, hungry or angry child, you'll lose.

Routine

Children need a certain amount of *routine* in their lives, so that they never get pushed past their body's refuelling needs. Put the child to bed *before* he cracks with tiredness. If he is angry, he needs time to cool off and often a face-saving way out of the conflict.

Handle conflict

What do we do when we find ourselves in the middle of a conflict situation? – *Withdraw*, either ourselves or the children. With a tiny child, withdrawing is easy, sometimes as simple as substituting a toy or moving the child away from the problem. Very little people respond well to distraction, but older children require stronger measures.

'No'

Don't say 'No' if you are going to change your mind down the track. 'No' *means* 'No' and 'Yes' *means* 'Yes'. Stick to your decisions, but listen to yourself. Are you giving mixed messages? Do you say 'No' when you really mean, 'If you put on a good enough tantrum, I'll change my mind?'

Whingeing

A child only whinges if whingeing works. You, as a parent, ask for what you get. If you reward a whinger by giving him what he whinges for, you are rewarding *unacceptable* behaviour. Instead, reward *acceptable* behaviour. Change it around. A reward doesn't have to be anything more than a quiet smile, a pat on the head, just some little acknowledgement that you've noticed how helpful or thoughtful the child has been; try it. It works on husbands and wives too!

Respond in the beginning

Be prepared to address the problem in the beginning, because you will have to address it in the end anyway and by then you will be angry.

It is *not* easier just to let something slip by, apparently unnoticed, because you feel too worn out to do anything about it. It is much harder the next time because children just get more and more 'hyped up' and harder to stop. Children often push hard to find out what the limits are and feel secure when they know where they fit in.

They know we always *love* them, but they have to earn the *liking*. Feel free to express this to them. Say something such as, 'I just don't like you when you do such and such; you know I always love you, but sometimes I really don't like you.'

Many parents say to me, 'Yes, but, he's got a cold' or 'He's only little' or 'She does not understand.' This tells you that the parents are not quite ready to face up to the problem. Point this out to them. Ask 'Is this perhaps *your* problem: are you afraid to appear too tough?', 'Are you trying to be the "nice" parent?' Give them time to talk about this. Parents will usually raise many family situations, often against each other. Don't allow 'nit-picking' or nastiness. You, the therapist, have to respond at the beginning to prevent unpleasantness from creeping in and to maintain your rapport with the parents.

The next step is to make sure that the child stops the unacceptable behaviour. If you have 'reacted in the beginning' and neither of you has become angry, it is just a matter of actually stopping or removing the problem. Do not leave the child at this stage in a confrontational frame of mind, distract him, start something new. Put your arm around his shoulders and walk into another room or outside and think of an activity the child may enjoy. Some mothers find this distracting step a bit daunting; they feel inadequate to think up an alternative in a split second. If you feel this way, sit down quietly and think up some suggestions beforehand. You can distract the child where he is, by suggesting a way to make the game he was playing more interesting and also more acceptable to those around him. For example, Peter might have been making little roads with his block or constructional toys and started throwing the blocks. The throwing must stop, but neither of you is yet angry. Stand up and say, 'No, no Peter, no throwing', and take him quickly to the place where the block landed. With your hand gently behind him, put your hand on his, pick up the block together and go back to where he was playing. Don't nag, just leave it at that. Then get down on all fours and make a bridge, reach for a car or truck; do something to introduce another idea or aspect into the game. As he starts to join in, gently back off. Your message is clear: 'I don't like you throwing blocks Peter, it is dangerous, but I still love you. It's OK to keep playing, but respect everyone around you.'

Withdraw

When things get totally out of control, we have to work out a way to withdraw the child or ourselves. I try to get the parents to work this through together while they are still with me. The parents must agree on the withdrawal place. The child is likely to cry when he is in this 'time-out' place, but as soon as the crying stops, look in and say, 'Good boy, you've stopped crying.' If he starts up again, withdraw from the place and repeat the procedure.

When he stops, walk in and with a big smile, go right up to him saying, 'Good boy, you've stopped crying.' Put your hands on him, stroke him, pat him, cuddle him, whatever he feels comfortable with. No child will run away if your response is positive.

If a small child resists by throwing himself on the floor, learn how to pick him up without hurting your back. Bend your knees, keep your back straight, pick up the child and put him on your knees, then straighten up and put the child face down over your hip, with his head down and face forward. The dangerous kicking legs will be out backwards, his hips will be behind you, his waist against yours and his shoulder girdle in front. The arms can reach and rake, but you will be able to control his body, usually with one arm around his torso, the other free. He will be able to lift his head to see where he is going and sum up what is happening. (With large children or teenagers, you cannot use this approach. Instead, you need to build mutual respect.)

Use body language

Explain how to use body language for emphasis. When they react in the beginning (of the possible confrontation), parents need to use body language to emphasise the point. If, when you say, 'Please don't do that Michael', the child just continues, do not raise your voice but achieve more emphasis by standing up, moving towards or putting a hand on the child and repeating your instructions. The child will immediately be surprised by the early intervention and will probably respond appropriately. If not, go to the next step.

Be dramatic and carry the child

Pick him up and march, with heavy show-off steps, towards the withdrawal room; the child will learn very quickly what that means. He may stop crying. If he does, stop very dramatically, look down at him and say, 'Oh, stopped crying, good boy' and change your grip. Either put him astride on your hip or turn him around, so that you can both look each other eye to eye – this is a loving cuddle position. Turn dramatically the opposite way and head back from whence you came. If the crying starts again, look surprised, say, 'Oh, crying again!' Place him back into the original position on your hip, spin around, and head back towards the withdrawal room. Unless he stops crying, put him inside and say, 'When you stop crying you can come out again.' Put on a big act of being angry, rush about looking very fierce, whereas in reality, because you reacted immediately, you have no need to be angry and are therefore very much in control.

Repair the damage

This step overlaps the previous one. After conflict, we need to 'make amends' or 'repair the damage'. We need the child to accept the responsibility. On the one hand we do not want to be over dramatic, for even tiny children need to 'save face', but on the other hand, we want to get the ' no-nonsense' message across.

Intervene and distract

Consider a few possible situations within families. One child bites another. Be quick with your actions and use gentle but firm words: 'No Richard, we don't bite.' Take hold of the child, quickly take it to the one who was injured, put the aggressor's hand on the injured spot and rub it, saying, 'Sorry Peter'; then turn the child away and start up something new, a new game.

If you walk away before diverting it, the child will probably bite or hit again. It is still a delicate situation, so definite intervention and a change in the way the game is played is called for. You need a little ingenuity.

Do not berate the child loudly for a long time. You have repaired the damage so get on with the day and leave it at that. The child has received a very clear message: 'No, we don't allow that sort of thing. We still love you. Try again, sweetheart, you can do it the right way.'

Take responsibility for our actions

This shows the child that you can trust him to take on the responsibility for his own actions.

A thwarted child will sometimes resort to drastic methods, for example vomiting, wetting or soiling himself. In such situations, the same rules apply. The child needs to take responsibility for his own actions. Remain calm and talk through the event, directing the restoration. We do not *make* children do what we want because we are bigger but steer them in the more acceptable way so that they can become responsible citizens.

Some children get too clever: they immediately smile and expect to be let out. Let them out, but only if they behave.

Try again and earn the right

If you feel that a long crying session will follow, build in a face-saving way out. Set the kitchen timer. Set it for five minutes – just long enough for the child to feel withdrawn – then pop your head in the door and say, 'Are you ready to *try again*?' You are putting the onus on him to take the responsibility for his own actions. He has to *earn the right* to come back out where everyone is and it is entirely up to him, *but* (and I think this is terribly important), do not waver and let him out early because you feel sorry for him, or he looks cute, or you kid yourself he does not understand; he will soon learn, particularly if you are consistent.

Work out ahead what is likely to happen in a therapy session. Many children prefer to be seen without their parents (McDerment, personal communication, 1997). Others do not mind whether their parents are there or not, and some very much want them there.

Explain to the accompanying parents how you propose to handle a tricky situation, so that they will be on your side. If the child will not leave his mother or allow you to handle him, then after a getting-to-know-you time, advise quite calmly, that, 'I'll have to send Mummy out and she can come back when you are quiet.' Give him a short time to digest this and then say to the mother, 'Please wait outside. When the child stops crying, and *I'm* ready, I'll call you back in.' *You* and not the mother are to judge when she is to come back. Have a chair ready outside for her to sit on. When you work with children who are expected to be unruly, it helps to have a trained co-worker or therapy aide who can look after the mother, get her a cup of tea and chat reassuringly to her so that she can return to the room as soon as requested. Mothers are often fragile and need to be cared for.

It is essential that the mother sees as much of the therapy as possible because she may become the child's best therapist in the long run, and she needs to learn just as much as the child.

There are many ways of withdrawing a child. A big, empty box can be placed in the corner of the room to withdraw him. An inflated car inner tube can be put in the bottom so that when the child is placed in the open box, the tube gently supports him in a comfortable flexed position. The objective is to prevent the child from seeing, from the withdrawal position, the effect that his behaviour or crying is having on those around him. Children are very astute; even children with a severe intellectual disability who see the result of their behaviour, will intensify this behaviour if they feel it will gain them attention.

Group therapy

In the foregoing section, individual therapy was discussed. Some children respond well in group therapy situations. In the playground, I have often removed the unruly disruptive child and pressed on with the group. If I have needed to withdraw a child, it is *I* who retrieves him rather than anyone else. A box in the playground is handy because it is put there for the sole purpose of behaviour correction.

Many other places can, of course, also be used for withdrawal.

Be consistent

Parents do their best, but best varies every day

Unless you are consistent, the previous steps will have been wasted.

If we are foolish enough to allow our child to go unrestrained in the car, our child is statistically much more likely to be badly injured or killed. Therefore, from the day an infant comes home from the hospital, it is 'belted up' safely in the car. It knows nothing else, it never occurs to it to complain. If you are inconsistent about the correct use of seat belts, you will always have a fight on your hands. Many parents already know this, and seat belts are not an issue. This is one area of your child's life where you are totally consistent; you can be just as consistent in any other behavioural area.

Listen to yourself. If you are a nagger, it means you are not consistent and the children know that they can choose whether or not they do what is required of them. Tell a child once, use a nice voice, remind him once, then mean what you say, for example, 'Jack, breakfast soon, you'd better get dressed' and a little later, 'How are you going Jack? I've got the bacon on, do you need any help with the buttons? I'm putting your breakfast on the table.' If he fails to materialise, put the food away. When he appears for school, undressed, put him, his clothes and his books into the car or near the front door so that he can still dress himself and get on with the day. You will need to do this only once or twice, especially if this is very new to him, but do not give up. Your word is law. Be very matter of fact, giving the impression that you expect him to comply and that you are still friends. Do not berate him.

Allow children to make mistakes

Most parents cannot bear to do this. If children forget their swimming costume or lunch, do not rush up to school with them. Let them do without. Let them learn by experiencing the consequences of their own actions. Be careful not to nag about it either. A simple, 'Oh! You forgot your lunch, you must be hungry. I'll hurry up dinner for you' will suffice.

If we always fill in the gaps for our children, they learn that if something goes wrong, Mum will fix it; they are not responsible. Children who learn this lesson can become over-dependent and irresponsible. Ask 'Is it my need to be needed?' Are we building young adults that will need *us* to nurture them? Be honest with yourself. Get on with your own life as well. If you would like to, get a job, paint a picture, learn a language, do Meals on Wheels, try to build time in your life so that you will not need the children as your reason to be alive. Of course, parents have to spend a lot of time with their children, especially in the early years, but as they gradually break away, let them go. Be proud of their ability to cope. Teach them by your actions that you *trust* them to go their own way and have *faith* in their ability to make good value judgements.

Let children grow emotionally

Let children grow emotionally as well as physically. Teach them to respect others' feelings, ideas and property by your actions towards them and towards outsiders and friends.

Why is it that we put on a good show for our friends but often not for those that matter most, namely our own children and partners? Friends come and go, but family is always family. Work on a loving, caring relationship because a little effort reaps such a wonderful reward. So many parents have come back to me and said, 'I had no idea our child was such a lovely person, and I could so easily have missed out on that relationship.'

Chapter 5
Food and Chemical Sensitivities

Jenny Bennett

In today's society, there are some highly reactive people who are sensitive to minute exposure to some foods or chemicals. Owing to an abnormal immune response and often a genetic predisposition, these people can react to fumes from pesticides, herbicides, fungicides, cigarettes, perfume, car exhaust, paint, colourings, flavourings or preservatives found in some foods or even a food in its natural state. Chemical sensitivity often comes about through overexposure to one or more of 100,000 chemicals in use today. Sensitivity to food and food additives can also cause many and varied symptoms. Some adults and children display numerous symptoms that mimic many illnesses, and the association with food and chemical exposure often goes unchecked.

Appropriate treatment or avoidance of the offending substance can lead to remarkable improvement in the quality of life for the person who is sensitive to foods and chemicals. 'Awareness' and knowing what to look for make life much easier for all concerned.

Research has revealed much about the causes of these reactions, but affected people have to learn to live as comfortably as possible. Once learned, these new ways become easy alternatives and eliminate the 'allergy stress' on the body. By eating the foods that are tolerated, obtaining organic foods if necessary, having a safe water supply, cleaning the home without chemicals and avoiding chemicals wherever possible, many people with allergies can lower their total load to a point of tolerance. The degree of intolerance will dictate the degree of avoidance needed. Many therapists now find that learning, co-ordination, speech and language, or behaviour-related problems lessen or even disappear after food and/or chemical intolerances have been eliminated.

My story

About 10 years ago, I was almost totally incapacitated by reactions. At this time, I can remember watching a television variety programme on which a disc jockey, who was a paraplegic, was a guest. He had produced a record using his beautifully rich speaking voice as a voice-over. In a moving way, he explained his inability to do most things, although he still had the ability to appreciate many day-to-day happenings. Each verse finished with the words, 'If I can do it, so can you.' When questioned at the end of his performance about his courage and wonderful attitude to life, he replied, 'I believe everyone has some kind of disability: it's just that you can see mine.'

There was I, unable to tolerate almost everything around me, foods and chemicals, and he was able to earn a living despite what must have been massive disabilities. *I felt more disabled than him.* The words, 'If I can do it, so can you' rang in my ears and were an inspiration to me.

With the help of a specialist in environmental illness, I decided there and then to read as much as possible about the cause and effect of what was happening to my body and mind. Because each individual is unique, I found that much of the treatment had to be carried out by the patient, with guidance from a specialist. I had undiagnosed multiple food and chemical sensitivities and was ill for about 30 years with many varied symptoms. I counted 72 allergy-related symptoms over the years, ranging from nausea, chronic rhinitis, asthma and diarrhoea to many other respiratory, ear, nose and throat symptoms. As well as these symptoms, gastrointestinal, musculoskeletal, cardiovascular and central nervous system reactions produced a totally miserable existence. This is why it is so important for parents to listen to their children when they complain of nausea or tiredness, especially after eating, or if they are just not coping at school.

From the age of about eight, over many years, symptoms accumulated until day-to-day situations that were mundane, simple, everyday tasks to 'normal' people – those not affected adversely by foods or chemicals – were causing me constant problems. I also had a short concentration span and was often unable to recall what had been said five minutes previously. After I became aware of the reasons for my symptoms and avoided the allergens responsible, the troublesome substances that were causing the allergic reactions, my health improved dramatically. The new ways, after I learned them, became automatic, like riding a bike.

The list of symptoms below shows that food and chemical sensitivities can mimic many illnesses. One allergen may cause many symptoms, and one symptom may be caused by any one of several allergens. Parents or health professionals may not recognise that these symptoms are associated with sensitivity in the particular child. This is why so many undetected illnesses develop into chronic complaints, often over years, the twentieth century having brought new technology and, with it, new problems.

Sensitivity symptoms

I have experienced or observed the following symptoms:

Skin

Flushing, hot flushes, warmth, coldness and tingling.

Ear, nose and throat

Nasal obstruction, sneezing, nasal itching, runny nose, postnasal drip, sore, dry or tickling throat, clearing throat, itchy palate, hoarseness, fullness, ringing in or popping of the ears, itching deep within the ears, earache with red or normal eardrums, loss of some tones, sounds seeming much louder, dizziness, vertigo and imbalance.

Eyes

Blurring, double or temporary loss of vision, spots before the eyes, pain in or behind the eyes, watery eyes, excessive tear secretion, eyes hurt by glare, eyelids twitching, drooping or swollen and redness or swelling of the lids.

Respiratory

Shortness of breath, tightness in the chest, a feeling of not enough air entering the lungs, wheezing cough and mucus formation in the bronchial tubes.

Cardiovascular

Pounding heart, increasing heart rate, skipped beats, flushing, hot flushes, pallor, warmth, coldness, tingling, redness or blueness of the hands, faintness and pain around the heart.

Gastrointestinal

Hunger, thirst, toothache, belching, retasting of foods, ulcer symptoms, nausea, vomiting, swallowing difficulty, cramps or diarrhoea.

Genitourinary

Frequent or urgent urination, inability to control the bladder, bedwetting and vaginal discharge.

Musculoskeletal

Fatigue, generalised muscle weakness and pain, joint pain or swelling with redness, stiffness, arthritis, chest pain, backache, neck muscle spasm, shoulder muscle spasm, limitation of movement and spastic symptoms.

Nervous

Headache, migraine, compulsive sleepiness, drowsiness, grogginess, confusion, dizziness, imbalance, slowness, sluggishness, dullness, lack of concentration, depression, crying, tension, anger, irritability, anxiety, panic, feeling stimulated, aggression, overactivity, feeling frightened, restlessness, feeling manic, hyperactivity with learning disability, jitteriness, convulsions, the head feeling full or enlarged, sensation of floating, poor memory, misreading or reading without comprehension, variation of penmanship, feeling separate or apart from others, amnesia for words, numbers or names, hallucinations, delusions, paranoia, stammering or stuttering, claustrophobia, paralysis, perceptual dysfunction and symptoms typical of intellectual disability.

Food

A child's health can improve dramatically once the offending substance has been eliminated, frequently giving him the incentive to comply with dietary or other measures to reinstate normality. Foods can alter behaviour in many ways, and temporary elimination of some foods (see Appendix 5) is not too difficult. It is often easier to eliminate foods than it is to deal with the behaviour problem itself. Avoidance of the intolerant food can eliminate the need for drug treatments that are prescribed for more serious reactions. It is quite exciting and satisfying to know that, by removing an intolerant food, you can help the child to lead a more normal life. If my problems had been diagnosed 20 to 30 years earlier, I could have avoided many symptoms and associated problems. Mine were undiagnosed sensitivities because, until recent times, this was a discounted or discredited area of medicine. The reactions were well known but the causes were not. Fortunately today, a doctor practising environmental medicine can guide sufferers to success.

Food intolerance

Food intolerance can cause either extremely severe or low-key cases of multiple sensitivity. Commercial products that cause reactions include commonly eaten foods such as:

- brightly coloured drinks
- ice lollies
- biscuits
- chocolate and other sugar-rich foods
- milk drinks, consumed continuously throughout the day and night
- wheat-based foods.

Wheat-based foods are often a cause of neurological disturbance.

Glue-ear, which frequently goes unnoticed, can cause impaired hearing and lead to learning difficulties. It may be associated with intolerance to foods such as wheat, all dairy products, including chocolate, oranges or artificial colourings, flavourings and preservatives.

The following symptoms are related to learning disabilities:

- hyperactivity (overactivity)
- hypoactivity (underactivity)

- fatigue
- vagueness
- lack of concentration
- lack of comprehension
- variations in handwriting
- poor memory.

Until the offending substances are identified and eliminated, parents cannot improve their child's behaviour or health.

Many manufacturers have responded to informed consumers' demand and changed to natural products or natural ingredients that contain no artificial colours, flavours or preservatives. Parents need to read labels and refer to *The New Additive Code Breaker* book (Hanssen, 1989), available through local libraries, for further information on food additives and their effect on the body.

Children can also be sensitive to medication (including fillers) and synthetic vitamin and mineral supplements. Challenge children with vitamins and introduce vitamins as you would a food to the diet. This is a simple and effective way to avoid hidden problems. Some people are sensitive to various brands, including those made from all natural ingredients, perhaps being sensitive to more than one component, such as yeast or soy, even though the vitamin is natural and has no added sugars, milk, derivatives, colours, flavours, gluten, etc. Reactions to a daily dose of all natural vitamins can be classic examples of masked sensitivity.

Look for *masking* effects. Masking occurs when a food that is consumed every day 'tops up' the system and feeds a craving. For example, the cup of tea or coffee for relieving a headache, a chocolate bar to relieve a craving for chocolate or sugar, or another drink for the alcoholic, producing the 'hair of the dog' effect, covers the problem only for a while. Elimination diets can help to *unmask* the problem.

Many people seem to tolerate a food or chemical when they are constantly exposed to it. An elimination diet is an excellent diagnostic tool in this case to identify the offending foods.

Food elimination

Wilson (personal communication 1993) has found, in over 20 years of working with children described in this book, that this method of food avoidance and menu planning is highly successful for many people.

The food elimination section in Appendix 5 can be used as a handout for families.

Organic foods

If severe food intolerance is suspected or found, buy certified organic food. Most people normally select their diets from a smorgasbord of processed foods that are high in fat, sugar and salt.

Some broccoli is sprayed up to 18 times before it is eaten, and wheat up to eight times after harvest, as well as being fumigated in the silo. The logical solution is to lower the total body load of these extra chemicals. Successful results are proof that the benefits far outweigh any time and effort involved. Substituting certified organic food can help to reduce health problems. I found that I could tolerate many more foods if the foods were free of sprayed chemicals.

Consider the organic food option especially if symptoms *persist* when dietary and other changes have failed.

Chemicals

Man-made chemicals are used in almost all aspects of our lives – we either inhale or ingest them. They are substances foreign to our bodies, and some people – those with chemical sensitivities – are severely affected. Some substances are potent poisons that affect the central nervous system, alter brain chemicals and produce abnormal reactions.

A mother who is unaware of the problem may experience years of unhappiness with a child. Instead of a bouncing, happy, healthy baby, there are many nights of broken sleep, unexplained screaming sessions and an unsettled child; this can lead to strain, stress and total misery. When the child reaches school age, the mother has a few hours free from the troublesome child and the problems are transferred to the teacher. At school, the child's behaviour may include hyperactivity, poor memory, vagueness, hearing difficulties, mumbled speech, illegible writing, inverted/rotated letters or numbers and many other learning difficulties. Acts of unprovoked aggression are difficult to explain; a food or chemical may be the cause. Children and adults can be bewildered by the inability to control their own devastating behaviour.

If teachers and parents become aware of some possible underlying causes, the child can be helped to gain a useful place in society. However, if these problems are neglected, they can cause a life of frustration and unhappiness for all concerned. This is tragic because some of these sensitivities can be avoided, even completely eliminated, if the allergen is removed from the diet.

Chemical intolerance

Challenging chemicals is also important. Sometimes it takes months or years for a masked allergy to dominate and it can often appear as a new symptom. For example, a child who has had eczema may develop asthma and no longer exhibit the signs of eczema; a child who gets headaches may have bouts of diarrhoea instead. The common belief is that a child has grown out of the eczema suffered as a baby, and the asthma that the child has developed may be emotional and nothing to do with the masked sensitivity. This common belief can be incorrect.

Food or chemical intolerance can often be the direct cause of an emotional response. To the casual observer, the emotional response seems to aggravate the symptoms, for example, headache and moodswings, or aggression and asthma. In this example, the headache and moodswings could be caused by one chemical, such as petrol fumes. The aggression and asthma could be caused by fresh paint fumes. Other examples of emotional responses include hyperactivity, kicking, hitting, biting, crying, depression and unexplained violent or subtle moodswings that will be familiar to the parents of children who are sensitive to food and chemicals.

Eliminating the cause can bring welcome relief to both children and those who care for them. For parents and therapists dealing with these children, awareness and observation are their best allies.

Chemical intolerance is insidious because chemicals (dust, moulds, pesticides, dry cleaning fluid and other chemical odours) can be absorbed through the skin, through the lungs and from the digestive tract, any tissue or organ of the body thus being affected.

Bathing and cleaning

People who cannot tolerate chemical cleaning aids need to find new ways of cleaning the home effectively. I have used the following inexpensive and simple alternative methods successfully for more than 10 years for my own family of five. For details of alternative products obtainable through Action Against Allergy [AAA], see References and recommended reading.

My approach was to eliminate all commercial cleaners from my home. When I looked under the sink and in the bathroom and laundry cupboards, the number of bottles and cans that I had accumulated amazed me. I now use only three products to clean my home.

- bicarbonate of soda (for example from a grocery store or swimming pool suppliers)
- white vinegar (labelled '*derived from cane sugar*', from a supermarket)
- pure laundry bar soap (refer to AAA).

There is a range of hypoallergenic products for less sensitive people. However, begin at this basic level because interactions tend to be complex and can confuse the issue. Wash the dishes with pure laundry bar soap. You can bathe and wash your hair with the same laundry bar soap.

For clothes in the washing machine, I use the following method. Place two bars of pure laundry bar soap in a 2-litre ice cream container of very hot water for several hours until the soap forms a 'gel'. Place the clothes in the washing machine, fill to the three-quarter mark with warm water and add the gel. Fill the machine up with hot water and start the cycle. If your water is hard, you may need two containers of gel.

Bicarbonate of soda is an excellent alternative to deodorant, but buy this from a pharmacy. Apply the powder with the fingertips to dampened underarms. If the skin is sensitive, dilute the bicarbonate. You can use bicarbonate to clean the shower, bath, handbasin and toilet. It is a gentle abrasive, does not scratch and works very well. Bicarbonate can also be used as a stain remover for clothes by wetting the soiled area and rubbing bicarbonate into the fabric. Leave for about one hour and handwash the spot with pure soap. The process can be repeated if the stain persists. To soak chemicals from new clothing, add one cup of white vinegar to a small basin of water: hot water for cotton garments, warm water for delicate fabrics and cold water for woollens. If the colour runs, rinse the clothing and soak in a half to one cup of salt in a small basin half filled with water to set the dye.

Clean mirrors and windows with white vinegar: dampen the cloth with the vinegar, apply to the area and then wipe off with a clean, dry, soft cloth.

Altering the home

Mattresses

To control or minimise the effects of the dustmite, use 100% cotton zip-on mattress covers, 100% cotton pillows and quilts, and polyester and cotton mattress protectors (all dacron-filled brands). Buy two, if it is easier. Wash and dry the covers, protectors and sheets each week. If necessary, the affected person can wear a 100% cotton tracksuit to bed for warmth. In colder climates, 100% woollen jumpers and socks may also be required. Refer to AAA for where these can be obtained.

Chemically sensitive persons should avoid synthetic mattresses; 100% cotton innerspring mattresses are available.

Removing carpet

Removing carpet and polishing floorboards brings a major improvement in many cases of dustmite and chemical sensitivity. Apply three or four coats of a clear water-based floor coating. This water-based product emits little or no odour, so that sensitive people can return to the room within hours instead of weeks. (With solvent-based coating, it usually takes two to three weeks before the floor ceases to emit fumes.)

Cotton rugs

Use 100% cotton rugs that are small enough to wash in a washing machine: they are practical and inexpensive. Lambswool rugs, 100% wool carpets and rugs are often mothproofed with chemicals and should not be used. Lambswool rugs harbour dustmite, but they can be washed and dried in the sun.

Damp dusting

Dust all washable surfaces with a *damp* cloth to reduce dust. There are no harmful cleaning fumes to produce symptoms.

Furniture polish

Use cold-pressed olive oil as furniture polish when necessary.

A day in the life of a child who is food- and chemical-sensitive

A child who is sensitive to food and chemicals can be overloaded. Finding and eliminating the causes can be a major contribution to better health. (Refer to AAA.)

Bedroom

The child sleeps on a dustmite-infested mattress (alive and dead dustmites both being active allergens). The bedding has been washed in chemically based and highly perfumed washing powder and fabric softener.

Bathroom

The child's first stop on waking is the toilet and bathroom. The potent chemicals often found here include air fresheners, toilet bowl deodorisers, aftershave lotion, perfumed soap and deodorant, perfumed toilet paper and perhaps fragrance wafting from Dad, Mum or an older sister's hairspray or perfume, nail polish remover and freshly applied nail polish.

Kitchen

The child then moves to the kitchen, where breakfast could be a glass of orange juice followed by cereal, for example, wheat (often a common cerebral allergen), rice or oats, to which milk and sugar are added. He may have an egg, or toast liberally covered with his favourite spread. Any of these foods could cause the child a problem. The air is heavy with cigarette smoke and the odour of smouldering cigarette butts. Perhaps a stray mosquito, fly or cockroach has just received a short, sharp shot of a chemical surface spray. Clothes may have been lovingly ironed with perfumed spray starch. Clothing still contains chemical residue from spray-on stain remover or may just be releasing highly perfumed washing powder.

Perfumes are used to disguise the offensive odour of chemicals and to leave an impression of freshness. (There are low or non-chemical brands available for those people with less sensitive reactions.)

Bus or car journey to school

The next move is to catch the bus, which usually emits thick black diesel fumes into the air (a major problem for most chemically sensitive people). Many such people relate the connection of diesel odour with their trip to school.

School

The child arrives at school. The classroom may have been cleaned early that morning with offending chemicals. Worse than that, it may have been laid with a brand new carpet. The synthetic carpet can give off chemical fumes, especially when gas heaters are operating.

In the past, unflued gas heaters in some schools have been a major source of indoor pollution. Common synthetic materials give off gas, and this process ('outgassing') can produce higher pollution levels indoors than out. The effect is compounded in modern, tightly sealed buildings designed to keep us warm in winter and cool in summer. The room may have been given its six-monthly or yearly application of pesticide. Potent, solvent-based, felt-tipped pens are usually present, and each table is issued with roneoed or photocopied work sheets, leaving a heavy odour of methylated spirits or toner. Again, both can be potent allergens for a sensitive child. Perfumed and non-perfumed erasers can also be trouble-some. The teacher arrives at the child's table to mark work. He or she could carry a strong odour of cigarette smoke that is absorbed and held by synthetic clothing, or be wearing aftershave or perfume and hairspray.

At this stage of the day, the chemically sensitive child could be feeling nause-ated and fatigued, both very common symptoms. He could have a moderate-to-severe headache and will probably not be working to the best of his ability. He could be hypoactive or, alternatively, hyperactive, metaphorically 'swinging from the lightshade'. Either way, the 'penalty' is often directed towards the child. He is either sent to the sick bay, placed on detention or sent to the corner for misbehav-iour. If the reasons for his symptoms are not detected, as they are often not, he just drifts along as the typical underachiever.

Lunchtime

Lunchbreak arrives, and the child eats bread and sandwich filling, both probably containing artificial colours, flavourings and preservatives. He may be drinking cordial and have purchased a highly coloured ice lolly or chocolate icecream from the canteen.

The child may eat or play near grass that has been sprayed. Chemical methods of grass edging or weeding are used at many schools, and the chemicals are some-times applied during the children's lunch hour!

In one lunchtime, a 'different' child could emerge, presenting a Jekyll and Hyde personality, familiar hyperactivity or physical and mental fatigue. He is unable to recall any previous lesson. (The recall is there only when the allergen is not. Information has usually been absorbed, but somehow the recall is affected while the offending allergen is present.)

Although fatigue at school is usually thought to result from a late night, the food consumed at the evening meal, or solvent-based felt-tipped pens used for colouring in after dinner, could cause central nervous system reactions such as overactivity, restlessness, poor writing for homework, reading without comprehension or misreading. These behaviours prevent the body from resting and leave the 'victim' awake for hours. The child who does eventually sleep may oversleep and awaken lethargic, unwell and unable to function.

The parents must find and eliminate the allergen(s) so that the child has a chance of working to maximum potential. An allergen eaten with the next meal will cause the symptoms to persist, and the reaction will be perpetuated.

Conclusion

Exposure to chemicals sometimes has devastating results. Children of average or above-average intelligence, who, in the right environment, would be high achievers, do not achieve when they are suffering symptoms similar to those mentioned in this chapter. Most educators are now caring and receptive to the increasing medical evidence available on the subject of environmental illness. Doctors who are skilled in this area can be a wonderful support to therapists and parents. Foods that these children can tolerate can be obtained, and there are suitable non-chemical substitutes and solutions for the problem areas discussed. Many families experience a feeling of relief and well-being when they apply the three simple, practical ways of avoidance: eating foods that are tolerated, having a safe water supply and cleaning the home without chemicals and avoiding chemicals wherever possible. The families have an opportunity to live comfortable, positive and qualitative lives, with children who can reach their full potential.

References and recommended reading

Bennett J (1993) *The Allergy Tuckerbox*. Recipes for people with food sensitivities. Available from
    Jenny Bennett, 19 Fiesta Crescent, Copacabana, NSW 2251, Australia.
Bennett J (1987) *The Allergy Survival Kit*. Available from Jenny Bennett, 19 Fiesta Crescent,
    Copacabana, NSW 2251, Australia.
Carson R (1963) *Silent Spring*. London: Hamilton.
Hanssen M (1989) *The New Additive Code Breaker*. Lothian.
Mackarness R (1977) *Not All in the Mind*. London: Pan.
Mackarness R (1980) *Chemical Victims*. London: Pan.
Minchin M (1986) *Food for Thought*. Melbourne: Unwin.
Randolph T (1981) *Allergies: Your Hidden Enemy*. New York: Wellingsborough Turnstone.
Rapp D (1991) *Is This Your Child? Discovering and Treating Unrecognised Allergies*. New York: William
    Morrow.
Verkerk R (1990) *Building out Termites*. Sydney: Pluto Press.

For further information on local brand names and outlets for alternative products, contact Action
Against Allergy, PO Box 278, Twickenham Middlesex TW1 4QQ UK. (0181 744 1171).

Appendix 1.1
Instruments for the assessment of children

Test	Birth to toddler	Preschool	Elementary	Mid-Primary	Upper Primary	Secondary	Adult
Screening Tests							
Capital Area Treatment Rating–CATR (Farley et al., 1991)		✓	✓	✓	✓	✓	✓
Infant/Toddler Screen for Everybaby–ITSE (Miller, 1993a)	✓	✓					
Infant/Toddler Symptom Checklist (DeGangi et al., 1995)	✓						
Scotopic Sensitivity/Irlen Syndrome Screen-SSIS (Irlen, 1991)				✓	✓	✓	✓
Miller Toddler and Infant Motor Evaluation–TIME (Miller, 1993b)	✓	✓					
Motor Developmental Checklist for Infants Stressed Prenatally with Maternal Cocaine use (Cratty, 1994)	✓						
NEED Screen (Edwards, 1980)		✓	✓	✓	✓	✓	
Quick Neurological Screening Test (Mooti et al., 1978)			✓				
Screening Test for Evaluating Preschoolers First STEP (Miller, 1992)		✓	✓				
Test of Sensory Functions in Infants TSFI (DeGangi and Greenspan, 1989)	✓						
Touch Inventory for Elementary School-aged Children–TIE (Royeen and Fortune, 1990)			✓				
Non-standardised Tests							
Clinical Observations (Wilson 1984)		✓	✓	✓			
Clinical Observations of Motor and Postural Skills – COMPS (Wilson et al., 1994)			✓	✓	✓		

Non-standardised Tests	Birth to toddler	Preschool	Elementary	Mid-Primary	Upper Primary	Secondary	Adult
Pediatric Clinical Tests of Sensory Interaction for Balance – P-CTSIB (Richardson *et al.*, 1992)		✓	✓	✓	✓		
Standardised Tests							
Bruininks-Oseretsky Test of Motor Proficiency – BOTMP (Bruininks, 1978)		✓	✓	✓	✓	✓	
Detroit Test of Learning Aptitude – Primary DTLA-P (Hammill and Bryant, 1986)		✓	✓	✓			
Goodenough – Harris Drawing Test (Goodenough and Harris, 1963)		✓	✓	✓	✓	✓	✓
McCarron Assessment of Neuromuscular Development–MAND (McCarron, 1982)		✓	✓	✓	✓	✓	✓
Miller Assessment for Preschoolers – MAP (Miller, 1988b)		✓	✓				
Movement Assessment Battery for Children – Movement ABC (Henderson and Sugden, 1992)		✓	✓	✓	✓		
Sensory Integration and Praxis Tests – SIPT (Ayres, 1989)		✓	✓	✓			
Southern California Postrotary Nystagmus Test – SCPNT (Ayres, 1975)		✓	✓	✓			
Southern California Sensory Integration Tests – SCSIT (Ayres, 1972b)		✓	✓	✓			
Additional Tests							
Developmental Test of Visual-Motor Integration – VMI (Beery, 1989)		✓	✓	✓	✓	✓	✓
Developmental Test of Visual Perception-2 – DTVP-2 (Hammill *et al.*, 1993)		✓	✓	✓			
Motor Free Visual Perception Test – MVPT (Colarusso and Hammill, 1972)		✓	✓	✓			
Test of Visual-Perceptual Skills (non-motor) - TVPs (Gardner, 1988)		✓	✓	✓	✓	✓	
Coopersmith Self Esteem Inventory: School Form (Coopersmith, 1981)				✓	✓	✓	
Piers - Harris Children's Self–concept Scale (Piers and Harris, 1984)			✓	✓	✓	✓	
Diagnosis and Remediation of Handwriting Problems – DRHP (Stott *et al.*, 1985)			✓	✓	✓	✓	
Handwriting Checklist (Alston and Taylor, 1984)						✓	
NEED Observation of Writing – NOW (Edwards, 1981)			✓	✓	✓	✓	

See Chapter 2 for references.

Appendix 1.2
Checklist: The child with learning and co-ordination problems

The child reveals some or any of the following:

- is poor at any of these – reading, spelling, maths, writing
- reverses letters and words
- has a short concentration span
- is easily distractible
- is one of the last to get books ready (does not seem 'to get his or her act together')
- has problems with keeping up with his peers in motor skills at pre-school level
- has poor co-ordination
- is slower at doing tasks
- trips over and/or bumps into objects
- cannot catch, throw or kick a ball well
- is very active or very placid
- has behaviour problems.

Birth history and milestones

(Milestones are the ages that children sat, rolled over, crawled, walked or ran.)

- Did not have history of problems during mother's pregnancy or at birth
- sometimes had early feeding problems
- sometimes cried a great deal, was irritable or fussy
- did not sleep much, slept badly or slept a great deal
- was active as a baby or as a young child
- was unusually placid as a baby
- motor and speech milestones were a little slow
- usually ran as soon as he or she walked
- climbed all over the place or was a late or non-climber
- took time to manage steps without a rail

- constantly fell over and into objects
- pushed tricycle with the feet; did not use the pedals.

Motor skills

Gross motor skills

- Catching – may be good, or poor if the child is clumsy
- throwing – may be hard or soft
- kicking – may have little or no sense of direction
- running – may have no problems or may be awkward
- skipping – may be difficult or impossible
- jumping with feet together – may be difficult, or the feet may be out of time
- hopping – may be awkward, or the child may hop only on one foot and not the other
- skipping with a rope – may be difficult and the child is awkward
- balancing – may be good, or poor if the child is clumsy.

Fine motor skills

- Colouring in – often difficult to stay within the lines
- cutting out – awkward or difficult
- pasting – often messy
- writing – poor; often uses primitive grasp; presses heavily; holds pencil tightly; poorly and immaturely formed letters; poor spacing
- managing or manipulating puzzles and constructional toys is difficult and therefore he or she loses interest

General

- Requires a great deal of concentration and effort to manage most of the fine motor activities
- may not know left from right
- may have no real hand preference
- may prefer the hand that is awkward to use and not the familial preference.

Dressing

- May put shoes on the wrong feet
- may have difficulty and/or take a long time to do up shoelaces
- may have difficulty with buttons and/or do up the wrong ones
- may be slow to learn buttoning
- may put clothes on back to front or inside out.

Eating

- Has difficulties with learning to use a knife and fork
- is a sloppy eater and often prefers to use his or her fingers
- may prefer soft food, which is easy to chew

- may chew with the mouth open (especially if he or she is a 'mouth breather')
- may be a messy eater
- has difficulties pouring a drink and then tends to spill it
- 'shakes' when carrying a cup, etc.

Communication

- Has problems remembering messages and following instructions unless they are very simple
- has a poor memory
- often 'tunes out'
- jumbles speech when he or she is excited
- can be very quiet or is a non-constructive chatterer
- has articulation problems
- mixes up syllables and words.

Play

- May prefer outdoor activities to indoor or vice versa
- flits from one activity to another although can stick to one thing if he or she is interested and can manage it
- has difficulty amusing him or herself.

Social and emotional skills

- Can be very active or can be shy, timid and quiet
- can be made fun of by peers because he or she cannot keep up with them
- may join in games with peers or else be a 'loner'
- opts out of and tends not to persevere with activities that he or she finds difficult
- can have difficulty coping with change in new situations
- tends to play with younger children
- has a short concentration span
- is easily distracted
- is good at manipulating people and situations to get out of things he or she finds difficult

Health

- Hearing – there is often an associated history of middle ear infections, requiring treatment with antibiotics
- vision – may cause associated visual co-ordination difficulties
- sensitivities to food and chemicals are sometimes present
- intelligence – normal; verbal scores are often considerably higher than performance scores
- physical appearance is normal.

Appendix 1.3
Occupational Therapy Parent Questionnaire

Identifying data

Child's name:
Date of birth:
Address:
Telephone:
Country of birth:

Reason for referral

Who suggested that your child should be assessed by an occupational therapist?

Why?

What do you feel are your child's main difficulties?

1. Family structure

Father's name:
Occupation:
Mother's name:
Occupation:
Siblings (brothers and sisters):
Parents' marital status:

Please indicate whether the parents are separated or divorced, and who is the child's legal guardian and has custody:

Do any family members have a learning or physical difficulty? (Please describe.)

2. Medical history

Local doctor:
Address:
Specialist(s):

Name:
Address:

Name:
Address:

Has your child suffered any illnesses or injuries? (Please describe.)

Has your child been admitted to hospital? (Please describe the child's age, reason for and length of stay.)

Please describe your child's general health.

Does your child suffer from any of the following?

	YES	NO	COMMENTS
Allergies			
Colds			
Ear infections			
Epileptic fits			
Car sickness			

Have the following been tested?

	YES	NO	WHEN	COMMENTS
Vision				
Hearing				

Has your child previously been assessed for or received occupational therapy? (Please describe.)

Has your child received any of the following services?

	YES	NO	PLEASE DESCRIBE
Speech and language therapy			
Physiotherapy			
Other			

Is your child under- or overweight?

Does your child have eating problems or any unusual food preferences? (Please describe.)

Do you have any concerns about your child's diet?

3. Child development

a) Early development

Pregnancy
Gestation period:
Medication:
Smoking:

Birth
Birth weight:
Health of mother at birth:
Any difficulties? (Please specify):

Feeding
Breast:
Bottle:
Any feeding difficulties? (e.g. sucking, swallowing or chewing):

b) General development

How do you feel your child developed compared with other children?

SKILL	EARLY	AVERAGE	LATE	COMMENT
Rolled over				
Sat				
Crawled				
Walked				
Played with toys				
Combined words				

4. Self-care

a) Feeding

How does your child:

SKILL	CANNOT	NEEDS HELP	INDEPENDENT	COMMENTS
Drink				
Feed				
Use a spoon				
Use a fork				
Use a knife				
Pour drinks				

b) Dressing

Can your child:

	YES	NO	COMMENTS
Undress			
Dress self			
Manage buttons			
Do up a zip			
Tie shoelaces			

c) Personal Care

Can your child:

	YES	NO	COMMENTS
Take self to the toilet			
Wash hands			
Shower/bath self			
Clean teeth			
Comb hair			

d) Toilet training

Age obtained bladder control:
Age obtained bowel control:

5. Gross motor skills

Does your child:

	YES	NO	COMMENTS
Fall or lose balance			
Appear clumsy			
Ride a two-wheeler bike			
Catch a ball well			
Throw a ball well			
Hop on either leg			

6. Fine motor skills

Does your child:

	YES	NO	COMMENTS
Prefer to use left/right hand			
Draw shapes (e.g. circles and squares)			
Cut with scissors			
Manage constructional games (e.g. Lego or jigsaws)			
Thread beads			
Colour within the lines			
Paste in without a mess			

7. Language and communication

Are you concerned about your child's skills in:

	YES	NO	COMMENTS
Being understood by others			
Following instructions			
Speech articulation			

Other concerns re communication skills:

8. Behaviour and concentration

Describe your child's behaviour at home.

Describe your child's relationship with other family members.

Are any of these problems with your child?

	YES	NO	COMMENTS
Overactive			
Irritable			
Aggressive			
Bad tempered			
Difficult to discipline			
Quiet			
Underactive			
Withdrawn			
Fussy			
Easily distracted			
Difficulty concentrating			
Wants to go to bed early			
Slow to go to sleep			
Enjoys being touched and cuddled			
Fearful of heights			
Fearless of climbing			
Memory			

9. Social and emotional skills

Is your child?

	YES	NO	COMMENTS
Friendly			
Easy going			
Talkative			
Nervous			
Shy			
Teased			

Does your child tease other children?

How does your child get on with:

a) other children
b) adults

Does your child lack self-confidence or have low self-esteem?

10. School performance

Present school:
Name of teacher:
Class:

Previous schools attended (including nursery school):
Please describe any difficulties experienced or classes repeated.

Describe your child's ability in the following:

(Rating scale: 1=poor, 2=fair, 3=average, 4=good, 5=excellent; circle appropriate number.)

	RATING	COMMENTS
Spelling	1 2 3 4 5	
Reading	1 2 3 4 5	
Mathematics	1 2 3 4 5	
Handwriting	1 2 3 4 5	
Other subjects	1 2 3 4 5	
Sport and gross motor skills	1 2 3 4 5	
Fine motor (manipulation) skills	1 2 3 4 5	
Behaviour in class	1 2 3 4 5	
Teacher's opinion of child's ability	1 2 3 4 5	

Do you want us to liaise with the school and/or send them a copy of the occupational therapy report? Yes/No.

11. General

When were you first aware that your child had a problem?

Who noticed it?

What do you feel may be the major contributing factor(s)?

Outline what others have said about your child's problem(s):

What are your child's assets/good points? (List at least three.)

What are your child's goals?

What are your goals for your child?

Do you have any further comments or concerns, including your opinion regarding the reason for this referral?

Please provide or attach any additional information that you feel will assist us in understanding and helping your child.

Questionnaire completed by:

Relationship to child:

Signature:

Date:

Acknowledgements

Occupational Therapy Department Westmead Hospital, Sydney, NSW, Australia.

Occupational Therapists: Gail Curby, Louise French, Lyn Lennox, Jennifer Shepherd, Elaine B. Wilson

Appendix 1.4
Sample letter to accompany School Questionnaire

Date:

Dear Principal/Teacher,

I am writing to ask you whether you would be kind enough to complete this questionnaire given to you by the parents of one of your students . . . . who is at your school. He/she was referred to our service for assessment on . . . .

The team aims to assist children who have co-ordination, language, behavioural, school and physical problems that may be affecting the child's learning ability, sporting skills, general social skills and confidence.

Your co-operation in supplying the enclosed information will be greatly appreciated. However, we respect the school's right to withhold information if desired. All information is confidential to the team.

I would be grateful if you could complete and return this form, either directly to me or to the parents, prior to the student's assessment date. I will forward you a copy of the assessment report if I have the parents' permission.

Please contact me with any enquiries you have regarding this referral or this service.

Thanking you.

Yours sincerely,

Occupational Therapist

Acknowledgement

Modification of letter sent by Jennifer Shepherd and Simone Kingsford-Smith, Occupational Therapists, Orana Community Health Centre, Dubbo, NSW, Australia.

Occupational Therapy School Questionnaire

Would the class teacher please complete this page:

Name of child: Date of birth:
Class: Teacher:
School:

What do you feel are the child's main problems, if any?

Do you have concerns about:
Vision?
Hearing?
Health problems?

Has the child's reading, spelling, number or writing scheme changed recently?

Results of any IQ tests:

Please describe any special help the child is presently receiving.
Please comment on availability of resources for special help (e.g. a support teacher).

Has the child been referred to any other agencies?

Child's assets (list at least three):

(Rating scale: 1=poor, 2=fair, 3=average, 4=good, 5=excellent; circle appropriate number)

		Scale	Comments
1.	**Learning skills**	1 2 3 4 5	
2.	**Memory**		
	recent recall	1 2 3 4 5	
	long term	1 2 3 4 5	
	remembers routines	1 2 3 4 5	
3.	**Reading skills**		
	knowledge of letter sounds	1 2 3 4 5	
	word attack skills	1 2 3 4 5	
	reading comprehension	1 2 3 4 5	
	speed of reading	1 2 3 4 5	
	overall reading skills	1 2 3 4 5	

		Scale	Comments
4.	**Spelling skills**	1 2 3 4 5	
5.	**Handwriting skills**		
	form of neatness	1 2 3 4 5	
	speed – keeping up with class	1 2 3 4 5	
	completing work	1 2 3 4 5	
	copying from blackboard	1 2 3 4 5	
	spacing between words	1 2 3 4 5	
	immature formation of letters	1 2 3 4 5	
6.	**Number/arithmetic skills**		
	basic operations – addition	1 2 3 4 5	
	– subtraction	1 2 3 4 5	
	– multiplication	1 2 3 4 5	
	– division	1 2 3 4 5	
	skills in use of abstract concepts	1 2 3 4 5	
	overall arithmetic/number skills	1 2 3 4 5	
7.	**Visual–perceptual skills**		
	visual perceptual skills overall	1 2 3 4 5	
8.	**Language and communication**		
	oral expression	1 2 3 4 5	
	written expression	1 2 3 4 5	
	clarity of speech/articulation	1 2 3 4 5	
	fluency – repetition/hesitation	1 2 3 4 5	
	vocabulary	1 2 3 4 5	
	language comprehension	1 2 3 4 5	
	follows directions given to class	1 2 3 4 5	
	follows directions given to individual	1 2 3 4 5	
	overall communication	1 2 3 4 5	
9.	**Physical skills**		
	gross motor (e.g. skip or hop)	1 2 3 4 5	
	skill in sports/ball games	1 2 3 4 5	
	fine motor	1 2 3 4 5	
	skills/manipulation (e.g. scissors and shoelaces)	1 2 3 4 5	
	preferred/established handedness	L/R/both	

	Scale	Comments
10. Development		
Emotional and personal		
self-esteem/confidence	1 2 3 4 5	
concentration/attention	1 2 3 4 5	
motivation in classroom work	1 2 3 4 5	
completes homework	1 2 3 4 5	
aggression	1 2 3 4 5	
Social		
gets on well with peers	1 2 3 4 5	
gets on well with adults	1 2 3 4 5	
withdrawn or isolated	1 2 3 4 5	
gets teased or bullied	1 2 3 4 5	
teases others or is spiteful	1 2 3 4 5	
plays with younger children	1 2 3 4 5	
classroom behaviour problems	1 2 3 4 5	
willingness to join in team games	1 2 3 4 5	

General comments and recommendations

Class teacher:

Support teacher:

School counsellor:

Please attach any relevant documents (e.g. school report and copies of writing, spelling, arithmetic and drawing).

Signature:

Position: Date:

Appendix 1.5
Screening guide for Irlen Syndrome

Ask the student with the help of the parents/teachers:

When reading do you:
- use your finger or something else as a marker, to keep your place
- lose your place without a guide
- skip whole lines
- skip words
- repeat lines
- reread in order to understand
- start off reading well, then slow down
- read a page and can't remember what you've read
- avoid reading when you can
- feel that your eyes are irritated by glossy paper
- find it is more comfortable to read on coloured paper
- read word by word
- stop and start
- feel sick, dizzy or bilious
- get aching/itchy/watery/gritty/sandy/stingy/red eyes
- find that the print goes blurry or fuzzy
- find that the print moves/swirls/shimmers/shakes/runs sideways/has rivers going through it/runs together/looks squashed/looks above or below the page
- find that the white stands out more than the black print
- find that the print is easier to read upside down.

With schoolwork generally, do you:
- move your eyes closer to, or further away from, your work
- frequently lose your place or make mistakes copying from the black/white board
- find that the overhead projector hurts your eyes or is hard to read from
- get headaches after a day's schoolwork
- rub your eyes a lot
- squint, blink or open your eyes wide
- squirm a lot or put your head at an awkward angle

- prefer to read or work in dim or little light
- find it hard to cut along a line
- get sleepy or tired from schoolwork more than others do.

General – do you:
- get a headache from glare or sunlight
- find that sunlight is 'too bright'
- find that fluorescent lighting is 'too bright'
- squint because light bothers you
- want to wear a hat or dark glasses because of the sun
- hear your teacher or parents say that your writing is poor
- find it difficult to stay on the line when your write
- find it hard to keep maths columns straight
- find it hard to look at a computer or TV screen
- find it hard to concentrate at school or watching TV
- find it hard to see or catch the ball in sport
- hold onto a rail when going up and down stairs
- bump into people, edges of furniture and other things without meaning to
- think you are clumsy

If the student says 'often' or 'sometimes' to three of these questions, he or she could by symptomatic of the Irlen syndrome and it is advisable to refer on to an Irlen consultant.

London
Sonia Dimont, 137 Bishop's Mansions, Stevenage Road, London SW6 6DX.
Tel: 0171-736-5752. Fax: 0171-371-8232
e-mail: dimont.irlen@virgin.net

North London
Ann Wright, 14 Homestead Paddock, Southgate. London N14 4AN.
Tel: 0181-364-8086

East Anglia
Ann Wright, 4 Park Farm Business Centre, Fornham St. Genevieve, Bury St. Edmunds. Suffolk IP28 6TS Tel/Fax: 01284-724301
Hm: 01284-728623

Kent
Don Riley, 17 Ashford Drive, Kingswood, Maidstone, Kent ME17 3PA
Tel/Fax: 01622-842764 e-mail:
101567.2412@compuserve.com

North West
Joan Hillary, Beacon Lodge, Macclesfield Road, Over Alderley, Macclesfield, Cheshire SK10 4UB Tel: 01625-583841 Fax: 01625-584441
e-mail: 106123.1264@compuserve.com

West Country and South Wales
Patricia Clayton, 123 High Street, Chard, Somerset TA20 1QT Tel/Fax: 01460-65555
e-mail: pclayton.edusult@irlen.demon.co.uk

Central England
Brenda Sharp, 4 Lovetts Close, Hinckley, Leicestershire LE10 OYH
Tel/Fax: 01455-6153-53

Yorkshire
Celia Stone, Woodhouse Grove School, Apperley Bridge, Bradford BD10 0NR
Tel/Fax: 01132-509150
e-mail: celia.stone@binternet.com

Scotland
Ann Peck
49A Lockharton Ave., Edinburgh EH514 1BB
Tel: 0131-443-0322 Fax: 0131-228-9185

Appendix 1.6
Occupational Therapy Referral Form

Client's name:

Address:

Telephone:

Date of birth:

Age:

Care giver's name:

Contact details:

School attended:

Diagnosis (if known):

Identified difficulties:

Services involved:

Additional comments:

Referred by:

Date:

Acknowledgement

Jennifer Shepherd, Simone Kingsford-Smith, Occupational Therapists, Orana Community Health Centre, Dubbo, NSW, Australia.

Appendix 1.7
Occupational Therapy Report (Sample)

Name:

Address:

Telephone:

Date of birth:

Date of assessment:

Age at assessment:

Local medical officer:

Teacher:

School and grade:

Reason for referral

.... was referred for occupational therapy assessment by
....
It seems that .... may be experiencing difficulty with

Background information

1) Family structure:
2) Medical history:
3) Child development:
4) Self-care skills:

5) Gross motor skills:

6) Fine motor skills:

7) Language and communication:

8) Behaviour and concentration:

9) Social and emotional skills:

10) School performance:

11) General:

Assessments administered and results

(Delete sections which are not applicable)

A.J. Ayres Clinical Observations

This test assesses the efficiency of function of a child's nervous system in relation to learning, co-ordination, language and behaviour.   demonstrated that he/she has achieved some good skills. Results indicated:

He/she did well in:

He/she revealed:
- ☐ Slightly low muscle tone.
- ☐ Slightly irregular eye movements, in particular . . . . . .
- ☐ Difficulty performing slow controlled movements.
- ☐ Difficulty planning and executing rapidly alternating forearm movements.
- ☐ Slightly irregular thumb–finger touching.
- ☐ Difficulty with planning unfamiliar movements, particularly without vision.
- ☐ Awkward bilateral motor co-ordination.
- ☐ Poor oral motor control (i.e. tongue to upper lip – this can relate to fine motor control or speech difficulties).
- ☐ Slight deficiency in equilibrium (balance) reactions, particularly when posturally challenged.
- ☐ Slight deficiency with co-contraction (simultaneous contraction of opposing muscle groups to elicit a rigid posture – basic to joint stability).
- ☐ Slight deficiency in protective extension reaction.
- ☐ Some evidence of slightly uncontrolled finger movements (choreoathetosis) when posturally stressed.
- ☐ Difficulty in maintaining/achieving a prone extension posture (i.e. lying on the tummy like a banana). This relates to movement/vestibular system functioning.
- ☐ Difficulty in maintaining/achieving a supine flexion posture (i.e. curled up like a ball). This relates to co-ordination.
- ☐ Evidence of baby reflexes not being fully integrated.

☐ Inability to assume/difficulty in maintaining a reflex inhibiting posture.
☐ Difficulty with gross motor skills, e.g.
☐ Difficulty with fine motor planning, e.g.
☐ Difficulty with gross motor planning, e.g.
☐ Difficulty with fine motor control, e.g.
☐ Gravitational insecurity (fearful when his/her feet are not on the ground).
☐ Tactile defensiveness (does not like to be touched unless it suits him/her).
☐ Posture was

Postrotary Nystagmus Test

This assesses the efficiency of processing of the vestibular (movement/balance) system and its influence on the areas of the brain involved in learning, co-ordination, speech and behaviour. . . . . 's response was negligible/hyporeactive/within normal limits/hyperreactive, indicating that this system may not be/is functioning at an optimum/adequate level.

Motor Free Visual Perception Test (Colarusso & Hammill)

This test assesses a child's ability to understand what he/she is seeing in terms of spatial relationships, visual discrimination, figure–ground, visual closure, and visual memory. . . . . achieved a score considered to be above/at/below that expected for his/her age group.

Developmental Test of Visual-Motor Integration (K.E. Beery)

This test assesses a child's ability to perceive visually and reproduce manually (draw) a two-dimensional symbol. . . . . achieved a score considered to be above/at/below that expected for his/her age group.

General observations during testing

. . . . participated well during the assessment.

Handwriting

. . . . wrote his/her name using an efficient/inefficient right/left dominant tripod/lateral pinch/dynamic tripod pencil grip.
He/she held the pencil close to the tip and pressed heavily when writing, which can cause . . . . 's thumb/hand/forearm to ache.

Drawing

. . . . drew a simple line/detailed picture of . . . .

Summary and recommendations

. . . .'s functional abilities include:

. . . . experiences difficulties with:

- Sensory integration, i.e. receiving and processing information from some of his/her seven senses (movement, touch, pressure, vision, hearing, taste and smell). The sensory information is not being processed accurately or efficiently. This in turn affects the efficiency of the brain's function because the brain depends on good sensory integration to function well. In other words, the areas of the brain that are involved in learning, co-ordination, language and behaviour are not working so efficiently.

As well as this, the quality of motor function (movement) will not be efficient, as demonstrated by:

- Visual perception skills – copying pictures, writing letters and numbers the correct way, and interpreting accurately what he/she sees – can be hard for him/her.
- Holding a pencil properly. Difficulty with pencil grip is often associated with low muscle tone and poor co-ordination.

I suggest that occupational therapy can assist . . . . with the above difficulties.

Occupational therapy can include:

1. Home programme
. . . .'s parents have been given a detailed programme of activities that can be carried out at home.

2. Attendance at occupational therapy treatment sessions at the . . . . Centre. Approximately . . . . weeks of occupational therapy, followed by a reassessment.

Prescribed activities for . . . . aim to improve:

- vestibular–proprioceptive (movement-pressure) and tactile processing
- muscle tone
- prone extension posture
- supine flexion posture
- bilateral function
- balance
- general co-ordination

- fine motor skills
- eye pursuits
- learning
- overactivity
- self-esteem
- bedwetting/soiling
- visual–perceptual and visual–motor integration skills.

I suggest that . . . . should try to learn spelling (arithmetic/times tables), reading out aloud, while bouncing on an inner tube, trampoline or his/her bed (or while marching). The multisensory input involved in this activity frequently assists learning.

At school, ... should benefit from sitting . . . . the blackboard, and placing what he is copying from (at his left/right hand side; in front of him).

Handwriting: I suggest that . . . . may benefit from:

- holding the pencil approximately 1 cm above the shaving mark
- remembering to move the thumb and fingers during writing as shown during assessment
- concentrating on sliding his/her forearm across the page from left to right (with the wrist and fingers relaxed), pivoting from the elbow
- altering his/her posture during writing, i.e. holding the head up and shifting weight so he/she leans on his/her right/left forearm
- writing with a piece of carpet placed under the page so that he/she will learn not to press too heavily and therefore use less effort (if he/she presses heavily, the pencil will puncture or tear the paper).
- writing using a 'special grip' on the pen/pencil, as trialled during the assessment.

. . . . may benefit from assessment with a speech therapist/psychologist/ paediatrician. Call . . . . to make arrangements for this.

Please contact me with any enquiries.

OCCUPATIONAL THERAPIST
c.c.file
Parents
School
Local Medical Officer

Acknowledgement

Compiled by Jennifer Shepherd and Simone Kingsford-Smith, Occupational Therapists, Orana Community Health Centre, Dubbo, NSW, Australia. Additions made by Elaine B. Wilson.

Appendix 1.8
Sample letter

PO Box 547
ARMIDALE NSW 2350

6th August 1997

Dear Jillian,

I have really enjoyed working with you over the past few weeks. I am writing to let you know how you got on in the activities we did at your house. You probably also want to know about what we plan to do next.

You did really well finding the hidden pictures. The 'going visiting' game was another one you had fun with. You seem to know your right hand from your left hand without any problems.

The block puzzles really made you think. You got nearly every one right. You lost some points on the puzzles because of the time.

When it comes to writing you really work hard. I think part of the problem is the way you hold your pen. At the moment you hold it like this.

 I would like you to try to change your pen position so that it looks more like this picture. This will take sometime to adjust. You and I will do some games together to practise it.

Trying to stand on one leg with your eyes open or closed is a bit of a pain. I really made you think when you had to copy the strange ways I sat.

I suggest we play some games together each week for the rest of the term. We will do such things as swinging in the hammock, zooming around on the scooter board and bouncing on the trampoline. I look forward to seeing you next week.

Kindest regards
Helen

Appendix 1.9
NEED Perceptual–Motor Checklist

SCR**N**EE**D**N	New England Educational Diagnostic Centre
	Perceptual–Motor Checklist
Name Age School Grade	
Person completing checklist Date	

Note: The items listed below have been identified as possible indicators of perceptual-motor difficulties. Place a tick [✓] next to any items that apply to the child. If five or more items are ticked, the child should be referred to an occupational therapist for more thorough investigation.

- ☐ Poor posture
- ☐ Carries body awkwardly when moving
- ☐ Trouble holding or maintaining balance
- ☐ Clumsy in activities requiring co-ordination
- ☐ Moves one side of the body more efficiently
- ☐ Cannot change direction quickly
- ☐ Difficulty hopping and skipping
- ☐ Bumps objects and other people accidentally
- ☐ Accident-prone
- ☐ Problem climbing stairs
- ☐ Clothes are often untidy
- ☐ Poor eye–hand co-ordination (e.g. catching balls)
- ☐ Difficulty distinguishing left from right
- ☐ Regularly reverses letters and/or numbers
- ☐ Problem copying from the blackboard
- ☐ Messy written work
- ☐ Short concentration span
- ☐ Daydreams a lot
- ☐ Follows verbal directions rather than written (or vice versa)
- ☐ Poor speech (e.g. too loud, too soft or slurred sounds)
- ☐ Hearing problems

Appendix 1.10
Part 1: Clinical Observations Test

Name: Age: Test date: yr   mo   dy
Parents: Birth date: yr   mo   dy
Address: Telephone:
                                               Referred by:
Familial handedness: Child's preferred hand: R L MIXED
                                               UL posture/grip of pen:

1. Hyperactive/distract: **2. Tactile defensiveness:**   **3. Muscle tone:**
3 – normal activity   3 – no response   * – hypertonic
2 – slt. hyperactive   2 – or ? response   3 – normal
1 – def. hyperactive   1 – 2 responses or def.   2 – slt. hypotonic
                                                                      1 – def. hypotonic
                                                                      R/L differences

4. Independent eye closure (optional):   **Look through kaleidoscope with**
   circle if adequate, cross if unable   R L   R L

5. Eye movements: **Across**   **Pursuits**   **Convergence**   **Quick**
                        midline   **in general**   **Localisation**
                        3 – normal   3 – normal   3 – normal   3 – normal
                        2 – slt. irreg 2 – slt. irreg 2 – slt. irreg   2 – slt. irreg
                        1 – def. poor   1 – def. poor   1 – def. poor   1 – def. poor

   R/L differences

6. Ability to perform   3 – smooth
   slow motions: 2 – slt. irregular
                                 1 – jerky, too fast

7. Diadokokinesia: **Right —— times**   **Left ——times**   **Both simult. ——**
   Number of times   3 – normal   3 – normal   3 – normal
   palms slap   2 – slt. deficiency   2 – slt. deficiency   2 – slt. deficiency
   thighs in 10 seconds 1 – def. poor   1 – def. poor   1 – def. poor

8. **Thumb–finger touching:**

	Right	Left	Both simult.	Sides (by ears)
	3 – normal	3 – normal	3 – normal	can do
	2 – slt. irreg	2 – slt. irreg	2 – slt. irreg	can't do
	1 – def. poor	1 – def. poor	1 – def. poor	

9. **Tongue-to-lip movement:**

Upper lip	Lower lip	Sides
3 – normal	3 – normal	3 – normal
2 – slt. irreg	2 – slt. irreg	2 – slt. irreg
1 – def. poor	1 – def. poor	1 – def. poor

10. **Co-contraction:**
Arm, shoulder, neck
3 – normal
2 – slt. deficiency
1 – def. deficiency

11. **Postural background movements:**
3 – normal
2 – slt. deficiency
1 – def. deficiency

12. **Equilibrium reactions:**

Upright kneeling	Quadruped	Long sitting
3–normal	3–normal	3–normal
2–slt. deficiency	2–slt. def	2–slt. deficiency
1–def. deficiency	1–def. def	1–def. deficiency

13. **Protective extension:**
3 – normal
2 – slt. deficiency
1 – def. deficiency

14. **Schilder's arm extension posture:**

Choreo-athetosis:	Postural changes in arms:	Trunk rotation:	Head resistance:	Discomfort:
3 – normal	3 – normal	3 – normal	3 – normal	3 – normal
2 – slight	2 – slight	2 – slight	2 – slight	2 – slights
1 – definite	1 – definite	1 – definite	1 – definite	1 – definite

R/L differences: Arms raised R L: Elbow hyperextension R L

15. **Prone extension posture:**
3 – holds 20 or more seconds with moderate exertion
2 – holds to 10 seconds, or 20 with great exertion
1 – unable, or holds 0–9 seconds

16. **Symmetrical TNR:**
quadrupedal, head
flexed and extended
3 – no change in joint flexion or extension
2 – slight change in joint position
1 – definite change in joint position

17. **Asymmetrical TNR:**
a) **quadruped position**
3 – no flexion on passive head turning
2 – slight flexion on passive head turning
1 – definite flexion on passive head turning

b) **reflex inhibiting posture**
3 – can assume and maintain balance
2 – can assume only with great difficulty
1 – cannot assume

**18. Flexed position
supine:**
3 – holds 20 or more seconds with moderate exertion or holds with slight resistance
2 – holds to 10 seconds, or to 20 seconds with great exertion: or holds but is unable to take resistance
1 – unable, or holds 0–9 seconds

**19. Gravitational insecurity
supine position:**
3 – normal
2 – slt. deficiency
1 – deficiency

20. Rolling:

21. Hopping:

22. Skipping:

23. Jumping with feet together:

24. Number of seconds standing on one leg: L   R

25. Marching on the spot:

26. Heel-toe walking along a line:

27. Scissor jump:

28. Unilateral scissor jump:

29. Posture:
a) Spine
b) Hip heights

(i) posterior view
(ii) side view

c) Scapulae
d) Feet
e) Toes

Prepared by Jan Johnson, Faculty Co-ordinating Committee, Sensory Integration International. Additions made by Elaine B. Wilson, Jennifer Shepherd, Occupational Therapists, Dubbo, NSW, Australia.

Acknowledgement

A. Jean Ayres, Ph.D, OTR.

Appendix 1.10
Part 2: Comments and Directions for Clinical Observations Test

Handedness

Compare familial handedness. Note any left-handers in family (direct – parent, grandparent, sibling; indirect – aunt, uncle, cousin).

Upper limb posture/grip of pen

Ask the child to write his name, copy a sentence and draw a person. The exercise is to note how he holds his pencil, how hard he presses on the page and whether he has dynamic hand movements. Note the movement of his arm when doing the test.

Hyperactivity and distractibility

Observe for this during testing of clinical observations; note the answers to the Parents' and School Questionnaires, and later in the treatment sessions.

Tactile defensiveness

Observe during testing of clinical observations and note the answers to the Parents' Questionnaire and later in treatment sessions when you are physically handling the child.

Muscle tone

Check for hyperextension in the elbow and wrist, and observe this later during treatment. Hold the child's arms out in front and note whether they feel floppy and automatically lower. All these are signs of low muscle tone. Should the muscle tone appear 'normal', perform continuous repetitive movements to test the elbow flexors and forearm pronators for hypertonus. Sit the child on the floor and ask him to cross his legs; check for difficulty or discomfort with this. Lie him on the floor and check for any 'catch' in his hip adductors, which would indicate probable hypertonus.

Independent eye closure

See whether the child can close either eye. The hypothesis is that the non-dominant hemisphere closes the eye more efficiently than the dominant hemisphere. This can be looked at in a cluster of symptoms for hemispheral dysfunction.

Eye movements

Use an interesting pencil or an appropriate object that is attractive to the child's eye. Hold it about 20–30 cm from the child's eye and slowly move the pencil diagonally, vertically and horizontally in a 'box and cross' pattern and in an arc. Observe tracking and midline problems (blinking, eyes jumping or momentarily looking away). Do this test without the child's glasses on, but be aware of any specific visual deficits, for example, squints. Hold the child's chin if necessary to keep his head steady.

Leave the eyes to rest for 10 seconds before testing for convergence. Hold the pencil about 20 cm in front of the child's nose and bring the pencil close to his eyes. For quick localisation, hold the pencil 30 cm in front of the child's shoulder, 45 degrees to the side, saying, 'Look at my pencil/tortoise [on the pencil end], look at my nose.' Repeat this 15 cm above the child's shoulder level and 15 cm below it, on both sides. Note overshooting or undershooting.

Ability to perform slow motions

Say, 'Watch me: don't go too fast and don't go too slowly, then do it with me'. Start with the shoulders abducted to 90 degrees and the hands touching the shoulders. Slowly extend the elbows, then flex the elbows and return the fingertips to touch the shoulders. Do this first bilaterally, then reciprocally and then unilaterally.

Diadokokinesia

These are rapid forearm movements. You and the child sit opposite each other, forearms resting on laps. Demonstrate rapid supination and pronation, then ask the child to imitate you and say, 'Do this carefully and fast.' Count the number of times the palms touch the thighs, i.e. pronation, in 10 seconds. Observe for execution of the pronated slaps and compare the left with right side scores.

Thumb–finger touching

Ask the child to touch each finger with his thumb, in sequence, from index to little, and then back in sequence to his index finger, repeating this three times. Observe speed, co-ordination and right/left differences. The sides test checks tactile/ kinaesthetic/proprioceptive awareness to note whether he is reliant on visual monitoring. You may also like to try him thumb-finger touching above his head.

Tongue-to-lip movements

Demonstrate slowly, movements of the tongue to the upper lip, the lower lip and the sides of the mouth and then ask the child to do the same. Observe co-ordination and the ability to do this.

Co-contraction

Stand and face the child. Say, 'Squeeze my thumbs; don't let me push you, don't let me pull you.' Push the child back and forth five or six times. Allow some elbow flexion and give the child a chance to build up tone. If the child does not seem to comprehend what is required, get him to do it on you and try to move your flexed elbows. For neck co-contraction, put your hands either side or on top of his head and say, 'Freeze like a statue' or 'Be as stiff as a stick.' Move his head back and forth or from side to side about five or six times. Do not expect as much of the neck muscles as you would of the arms. This also tests co-contraction of the trunk and the lower limbs.

Postural background movements

Observe these body righting movements and postural adjustments during testing. Observe how easily the child adjusts his posture to complete a task. Does he shift his posture to avoid crossing the midline of his body?

Equilibrium reactions

Place the child in the positions stated (upright kneeling; hands and knees; long sitting with arms out straight in front of him) and say, 'I'm going to move you; let me move you but don't fall over.' Note the reactions.

Protective extension

Have the child in an upright kneeling position and then push him unexpectedly forwards, to either side and backwards. Note whether his arms extend well when he falls.

Schilder's arm extension posture

a) Say to the child, 'Put your feet together, arms out straight in front of you, spread your fingers apart, and close your eyes. Count up to 20.' Observe whether choreoathetoid movements are present, the child hyperextends his elbows or tries to stabilise his trunk with his hands together. Check whether the arms rise or lower.

b) After counting to 20, tell the child to keep his arms in front of him, while you move his head. Observe for arms lowering, arms following trunk, or resistance to head turning. Note any right/left differences.

Prone extension posture

Ask the child to assume the following position. The child lies prone, arms abducted to 90 degrees, elbows flexed, legs extended and not touching the floor. Demonstrate and/or place him in this position if necessary. If positioning or demonstration is needed, allow the child to rest and then resume the position. Have him count to 20 out loud so that he does not get a stabilising effect by holding his breath. Time it for 20 seconds because he is not counting to time. When he is in the position, slide a piece of paper under his thighs.

Symmetrical tonic neck reflex (STNR)

The child goes onto his hands and knees. Flex and extend his neck and observe for changes in joint position of elbows and hips and trunk posture.

Asymmetrical tonic neck reflex (ATNR)

a) Put the child in the hands-and-knees position. His head must be horizontal. Make sure that his elbows are not locked. Turn his head to the right and to the left and observe the amount of elbow flexion as the head is turned.
b) Place the child in the reverse ATNR position (hand on the hip, opposite leg raised and extended, head turned towards the side of the flexed arm). Observe the effect of the ATNR on equilibrium, noting whether the child can assume and maintain the posture.

Supine flexion

Ask the child to assume the relevant position or place him in it (arms crossed on the chest, ankles crossed, and flexion at the neck, hips and knees). Observe how long and how well the child can maintain the position. Count for 20 seconds. Let him rest then ask him to re-assume the position, while you apply resistance at the head and knees ('push him apart') and see whether he can hold it for you. The child does not count.

Gravitational insecurity

This is carried out at the end of the clinical observations because, if he is gravitationally insecure, you may 'lose' him. Test the child by having him sit on an unstable surface (a ball or tilt board). Move the surface. Stabilise the child by his ankles and knees. **You must hold onto the child**. Then ask the child to lie down backwards. He should be able to do this. Hold the child's knees and the board tilts as he lies down. Note the degree of fearfulness and necessity in changing the centre of gravity. Look at his face and listen to what he says.

Rolling

The child lies on the floor and rolls over and over. Is he rolling crookedly or stiffly? Does he 'hump' his bottom and not have a good segmental rolling pattern?

Hopping

Compare the difference in his ability to hop on each foot. Which leg does he commence with? Does he overbalance?

Skipping

Note his ability to skip. Can he do it first time or only after he is shown how to skip?

Jumping with feet together

Is his jumping in control? Do both feet hit the floor at exactly the same time?

Standing on one leg

Time how long he can stand on each foot.

Marching on the spot

Get him to march on the spot, swinging his arms, 'like a soldier'. Look for a correct reciprocal pattern.

Heel-toe walking

Get him to put his front heel right against his back toes along a line on the floor. Do this for 5 to 10 metres.

Scissor jump

Have him stand in a reciprocal position (e.g. right arm forwards, left leg backwards). Jump and reverse the positions. Note his ability to motor plan.

Unilateral scissor jump

This is the same as the 'scissor jump', but it is done with the same arm and leg.

Posture

Look at the child's posture with his shirt off. Check that his vertebral column is straight. Look at his scapulae (often winged). Look for a pelvic tilt and assess the level of his hips. Look at his feet: often flat. All these can be associated with low muscle tone.

Appendix 1.11
NEED Centre
Observation of Writing

N̄EED Centre
Ōbservation of
W̄riting

Name: Test date: /   /   Test age: /   /
Examiner: Writing instrument: ☐ pencil ☐ biro ☐ pen

Letter formation

Instruction: *Sit comfortably, hold your pen in your normal writing position, write in your best handwriting the small letters of the alphabet.*

Shape: a b c d e f g h i j k l m n o p q r s t u v w x y z

Rotations:

Posture

Instructions: *Write a few sentences in your best handwriting.*

Joint angles: ankles =   °   knees =   °   legs =   °
                shoulders =   °   elbows =   °   wrist =   °

☐ Postural adjustments (avoids crossing midline) ☐ Associated movements ☐ Repositions paper

Grasp

(Observe finger and thumb positions and identify writing action from the grasps illustrated below. Modify drawing to indicate specific features.)

Writing pressure: ☐ average   ☐ too heavy   ☐ too light

Letter formation at speed
Instructions: *Now write the same sentences as quickly as possible.*

Time (secs)   Number of letters   Letters per minute
Writing appears spontaneous: ☐ yes ☐ no Hand and finger movements
co-ordinated: ☐ yes ☐ no Faults not seen at slower speed.

shape   a b c d e f g h i j k l m n o p q r s t u v w x y z
rotation   a b c d e f g h i j k l m n o p q r s t u v w x y z
joints

Additional comments:

Adapted from Phillips (1976), see Chapter 2. Reproduced with kind permission of the NEED Centre, Armidale, Australia.

Appendix 2
Activities for sensory integrative treatment procedures

Vestibular-proprioceptive

- Lie prone/supine or sit, with a sheepskin rug, in the net. An inner tube can be placed in the net and the child sits on this. A ball can be placed in the net, which is threaded through the centre of a small inner tube before the net is suspended thereby having the inner tube outside the net but resting on the ball inside; a child can sit on this ball. Two children can sit in the net back to back.
- Lie prone/supine, sit or kneel on the scooter board going down the ramp.
- Lie prone on the scooter board and orbit or spin on the floor.
- Sit and swing in a vertically suspended tyre.
- Sit on a Sit'n'spin (you can tell the child to 'drive the truck'). The child can have his legs extended on a scooter board, which goes around as he turns the sit'n'spin.
- Have the child lie or sit and spin himself on the postrotary nystagmus board.
- Jump on or straddle and bounce around a tractor inner tube.
- Do somersaults over a large therapy ball and fall into a large pillow.
- Orbit or spin, sitting on a four-rope platform swing.
- 'Tarzan' swing on a suspended rope and jump from a table or chair into a large pillow.
- Sit and spin on a cable reel, either pushed by hand or spun around by someone pulling on a rope attached to the reel.
- Lie prone, supine or sit in the centre and straddle the bolster swing, with or without the arms out. Movement of the bolster can be back and forth or in an orbit.
- Kneel on a scooter board and pull on the net; go back and forth.
- Sit on a cable reel or scooter board; hold onto the bolster swing or four-rope swing and zoom back and forth underneath.
- Hold a suspended net and orbit around a pillow; the child can spin while holding the suspended net.

- Roll in five car inner tubes on the floor or down a ramp.
- Sit and swing in a suspended small inner tube.
- Lie supine on a scooter board and cling onto a small suspended inner tube with legs. Spin around on the scooter board.
- Lie prone on a scooter board, with knees flexed and legs hooked into a hoop, while you pull child around by the hoop.

Tactile

- Crawl up a ramp on the stomach and collect articles at the top. This can be a competition between two children. The child can crawl and push the scooter board up the ramp with his head.
- Pretend to be animals (duck, crab, seal, bucking donkey or frog) on the carpet.
- Crawl through or lie in the net or inner tubes, or roll along the floor in a towel tunnel. Lie in the towel tunnel, prone or supine, on the scooter board and be pulled around.
- Tumble onto a large foam pillow.
- Crawl under a large foam pillow.
- Use all the activities on any parts of the floor or equipment which are covered with carpet.
- Climb up a rope.
- Tug o'war.
- Lie in the net prone and pick up beanbags from the carpet.

Tone

- Jump on the inner tube while you press on child's head or shoulders.
- Cling to the underside of a bolster swing as it is being moved vigorously.
- Tug o'war.
- Sit on a space hopper, go down the ramp and crash into a large pillow. Hop along a coloured line on the floor.
- Climb up a rope.
- Play speedball.
- Jump with the feet together and zig-zag along a line.
- Walk along a line with a book on the head.
- Lie prone on a scooter board and hold onto a towel while being pulled around.
- Walk along an inverted reel and hold onto a suspended rope.
- Bounce around a tube while holding the rope.
- Tap around the mouth/cheeks and press the lips together to build up oral tone.

Bilateral activities

Upper limbs

- Hit a ball with a rolling pin or rod, while standing, sitting or lying prone on an inner tube, or standing on cable reel or tractor inner tube.

- Play speedball with the arms.
- Hit a suspended small inner tube with a rolling pin. Two children also can hit back and forth to each other.
- Throw a tennis or squash ball against the wall or up in the air and catch it with a bilateral cup. Catch beanbags in a bilateral cup. Do the above while walking around a tractor inner tube.
- Bounce on a large inner tube and hit a suspended tyre with a stick.
- Clean the board with two dusters using two hands.
- Straddle the inner tube or bolster swing and 'row the boat' using a broom handle held in both hands.

Lower limbs

- Jump with the feet together holding a ball/soft toy/animal/balloon/towel roll held between ankles. Jump either side of a line/along a coloured line/on Twister spots/between horizontally spaced straws, or do one jump, then two jumps, then three jumps, etc. in a zig-zag fashion.
- Play speedball with the feet.
- Play hopscotch with the feet together.
- Lie supine and hit a suspended ball with the feet together.

Prone extension

- Lie prone on a scooter board and go down the ramp with a soft toy on the back of the thighs. Tell the child not to drop this toy, so his legs will keep together.
- Push off from the wall and catch a ball.
- Lie prone on a scooter board and 'ford the river'. The child pulls himself across the 'river' by means of a rope hung from one side of the room to the other.
- Lie on a cable reel or a large inner tube and catch a ball or hit a ball with a stick.
- Lie prone on a scooter board and orbit, holding a hoop, which is pulled around.
- Lie prone on the floor and play speedball.
- Lie prone in the net with or without a small tube on the feet and neck to maintain posture, and pull on a towel.
- Lie prone in a net and catch a ball, animal or spider ball, or hit a ball with a rolling pin.

Supine flexion

- Lie supine and go down a ramp on a scooter board, catching a ball between the knees.
- Cling onto a bolster swing from the top or from underneath. Older children enjoy having a therapy ball tossed at them while they hold on in this position: it provides an extra challenge. Older children can have a competition and be timed while clinging on.

- Lie supine on a scooter board in a towel tunnel, orbiting, as you pull the child around.
- Lie supine on a scooter board, holding onto the bolster swing and moving back and forth. Hold onto a net and zoom; go through chair or table legs, feet first. Zoom back and forth between your legs while being held by the hands.
- Lie supine on a scooter board and 'ford the river'. The child pulls himself across the 'river' by means of a rope hung from one side of the room to the other.
- Lie supine, using speedball.
- Lie supine in a net, pulling on a towel.
- Lie supine on the floor and catch a ball or hit it with a stick.
- Lie supine throwing beanbags through a hoop.

Balance and trunk rotation

- Catch a ball while standing on a balance or nystagmus board.
- Stand on a side-turned cable reel and walk back and forth at first; then catch balls or hit a ball with a stick.
- Walk around large inner tube, catch a ball or play 'traffic lights' with red, orange and green coloured balls.
- Walk on two scooter boards on the carpet.
- Sit on a bolster swing with the arms abducted or with the arms forward. Upgrade this to kneeling and then to standing.
- Walk around a large inner tube and bounce a ball on the floor inside the tube.
- Kneel or sit on a scooter board with the hands above the head. Go down the ramp.
- Walk on 'feet' painted around a tractor tyre.
- Walk around a tractor tyre, one foot in front of the other, or walk backwards and change direction.
- Walk on stilt blocks.
- Hop along a line or on Twister spots.
- Walk cross-legged along a line, first forwards and then backwards.
- Stand on a balance board and throw a ball onto a Velcro dartboard or stickball.
- Kneel upright on a bolster swing and hit a ball with a rolling pin.
- Walk cross-legged on Twister spots, for trunk rotation.
- Roll along a line on the floor.
- Roll on the floor and collect and place quoits on pegs. Any articles or toys can be used.
- Rotate the body on balance or nystagmus board and play stickball.

Crossing the midline

- Stand on a balance board and hold two half detergent bottles. With the child's arms first apart and then crossed, throw matchboxes or beanbags into two half detergent bottles.

- Hold a stick vertically with both hands (with/without a sink plunger on the end). Jump either side of a line and, each time, place the stick opposite the feet.
- Stand on or off a balance board, playing 'Simon says' involving crossing-the-midline postures.
- Hit a ball (which is thrown in all directions) with a horizontal broom stick and move the arms across the body.
- Hold a rolling pin by one end, with two hands on that end, and hit a suspended inner tube.
- Straddle a bolster swing and 'paddle' the bolster back and forth, either side, with a long stick (both hands being held together high up on the stick).
- Lie prone on a scooter board, holding a stick with two hands, and be pulled round room.

Unilateral activities

- Throw a ball against the wall and catch it in a half-detergent bottle held in the appropriate hand.
- Hit a suspended inner tube with a rolling pin in one hand.
- Catch the ball in a cone.
- Kick a suspended inner tube with the appropriate foot.
- Jump on the tractor inner tube with the appropriate foot and fall onto that side onto the pillow.
- Hop along a coloured line with or without a small beanbag under the foot.

Protective extension

- Lie prone, inverted across a bolster swing, leaning and pushing on the hands.
- Fall onto Twister spots. Tell the child which colour to fall on and hold the 'good' arm so that the child uses the other one while falling.
- Lie over a therapy ball and roll right over and down until the hands touch the floor.

Eye tracking

- Follow with the eyes two different coloured blocks in your hand and name the colour of the block being shown at that time. Rotate your forearm to switch the blocks and then have the child name the new colour.
- Follow the coloured ball as it moves in a 'box and cross' path.
- Follow your torch light track, you and the child both having a torch.

Eye–hand co-ordination

- Throw quoits, a frisbee or skimmer rings through a suspended tyre.
- Play Velcro darts or stickball.
- Jump on a car inner tube and throw quoits.

- Bounce on an inner tube, throwing beanbags into circles or boxes.
- Catch animals on the flexor swing.

Motor planning

- Jump in patterns on the Twister sheet.
- Follow instructions written on cards.
- Jump, bounce a ball, jump, throw a ball and catch it, and so on.
- Lie prone on a scooter board and keep only one wheel on a coloured line.
- Walk cross-legged or one foot in front of the other, forwards then backwards, along a line. Take one step, twist the body and jump right around, take another step and so on.
- Jump on a space hopper along a line, forward two, then back one.
- Kneel on a scooter board and ride backwards.
- Stand on a tractor inner tube that has a reel inside it. Walk around the inner tube with one foot on the reel and one foot on the inner tube.
- Catch and throw a ball, clapping or twisting hands in between each catch.
- Manoeuvre a tractor inner tube by sitting on it in the vertical position and moving it along a path.
- Have a car inner tube race, each child rolling an inner tube vertically. One child alone can roll two vertical tubes at the same time.
- Bounce a ball over a rope or a bolster swing.
- Balance on a board and throw a ball through the hole in a suspended tyre.
- Bounce or pat a ball along a rope path.
- Get out of the towel tunnel without using the hands.
- Move slowly like a cat stalking its prey.
- Walk like a duck, crab, seal, toy soldier, bucking donkey, frog or pirate.
- Jump, hop, jump, hop along a rope path.
- Walk on felt or rubber footsteps in a forward direction, then backwards, then forwards again. Bounce a ball between each step.
- Have three people stand in a circle, two balls being thrown simultaneously.

Visual space perception

- Crawl through the legs of a ramp, head first, then feet first, in supine and prone postures, without touching any part of the ramp.
- Lie supine and then prone on a scooter board, and crawl through table or chair legs without touching them.
- Bend or scoot under a rope bar.
- Lie prone on a scooter board and perform a figure-of-eight around two chairs. Then do this with a paper bag on the child's head.
- Walk on a rope path that is on the Twister sheet.
- Have an obstacle course through table or chair legs, through an inner tube, under a sheet, through five inner tubes and through a tunnel. Pick up a quoit,

go through the hoop, put the quoit on the peg and do a somersault onto the pillow. (This is also a motor planning activity.)

Hyperactivity

Before starting the session, 'contract' with the child what he will do by listing or drawing the activities on the blackboard. As each activity is completed, rub that one off. If the child 'strays' onto something else, remind him firmly that 'We agreed to do ...'.

- Swing slowly in a regular net or a large hammock with a sheepskin, lying prone or supine, or sitting cross-legged. Hold the child firmly as he is moved.
- Do slow motor planning: 'Angels in the snow'. Here the child lies on his back and you stand and face him. The child follows your movements which are slow, for example an arm moving slowly out to the side, or a leg moving slowly forwards.
- Stroke firmly down and either side of the vertebral column with your index and middle fingers, one hand after the other.
- Lie the child on a bolster swing and give him firm touch pressure.
- Invert the child across a bolster swing, his head hanging down.
- Brush the child's forehead either side of the midline 10 times with a soft paint brush.
- Watch an egg-timer, or two different coloured egg-timers, while being rocked gently. Any fascinating activity that he can watch can be effective.
- Have a 'good behaviour' chart. Some children respond well to this.

Appendix 3
Home Programme

The home programme is a particularly important tool for parents who cannot bring their children in for treatment. It is *vital* that you use your clinical judgement to ascertain whether it would be appropriate for a particular family to follow this treatment regime and whether you consider that *suspended equipment* would be advisable for them to use.

Have a standard list of activities, *the appropriate ones being ticked after you have assessed the child. Before providing a home programme, always try the child out on the equipment to check his reaction to the activity and show the parents what is required.* It is extremely important to limit the number of activities suggested, so that the parents are not overwhelmed, but select alternatives that are manageable in the home and will keep the child interested. Parents should not force the child to do the activities because then they are less beneficial.

The home programme can be carried out for about 30 to 40 minutes, depending on the time that the parents and child have available. If there is time after school, it can be beneficial before the commencement of homework. This can be done daily (with shorter sessions) or three times a week. There may be time only at the weekend if it is not possible during the week. It is vital that parents co-operate willingly and that children enjoy the activities. Home programmes can be very successful if the father or an older sibling can assist; children love their involvement. If the child loses interest, recommend a break for about six weeks or suggest some new activities for the parents to instigate.

It is best that the child works in bare feet.

Endeavour to suggest activities that are inexpensive to set up at home.

Gross and fine motor, and gross and fine visual space perception activities are taken from the list of the typical treatment session in Chapter 3. Numerous gross motor activities can be given, or the parents can invent some. Tick the boxes beside the activities that you want the parents to employ. Any of the gross visual space activities can create an obstacle course. Include motor planning activities and/or the visual space perception games that have motor planning components, because both motor planning and visual space perception interrelate.

Sometimes you are limited only to providing activities that the child does himself without involving the parents. This may be necessary for working parents, single parents, parents who have commitments to other children, or parents who are unwilling to devote time to a home programme, but will set it up for the child to do it himself. It may be necessary also when the home programme is ongoing for a child who requires sensory stimulation, or when the child prefers to work alone.

Equipment

The following items of equipment, all of which can be obtained easily and cheaply, will usually suffice:

- a net hammock (provided or purchased at an army surplus store, suspend it from a tree, carport or suitable hook attachment)
- a car tyre suspended horizontally or vertically. The horizontal tyre is suspended by four ropes, attached to the tyre with four eyebolts and secured in the tyre by drilling holes in it or just through holes drilled in the tyre. The vertical tyre is suspended in a similar way but with just one eyebolt or hole with a rope through it. Wrap a small blanket or towel around where the child lies because the bare tyre may hurt him. Details of making these are in Appendix 4
- a truck inner tube suspended vertically with a piece of rope around it
- a ball
- a rolling pin
- a tractor or car inner tube, a mini-trampoline (jogger) or a trampoline
- a sheet or rug
- toys
- an icecream bucket
- small beanbags (50 mm × 50 mm) filled with rice; full match boxes, taped closed
- insulation tape for the floor
- a scooter board (from 0.3 m × 0.45 m up to 0.4 m × 0.6 m) with two pairs of castors on plates screwed on to the scooter board 50 mm in from the edge
- a piece of rope
- a bath towel
- two can stilts
- a blanket.

The following home programme can be reproduced and given to parents. Recommend that the child works in bare feet.

Home programme for you to use with your child

Keep in contact with your child's occupational therapist, who will keep progress notes and provide additional ideas if you need them. She will review your child after three months.

When your child is in the net hammock or the tyre, change the direction of movement every 30 seconds to obtain maximum benefit from this activity.

Your child must guide you in what he wants therapeutically. If he wants to spin or orbit in the net more, and he is tolerating the movement, allow him to continue. This is how he retains control.

If your child feels nauseated or dizzy, stop the activity *immediately*. If the sensation persists, massage the base of the skull, tell him to breathe in and out deeply or get him to push with his head against a cushion that you hold.

If your child becomes overactive, hug him and sit him on your lap while you rock him. Alternatively, include some of the fine motor activities while you rock him. The ways of calming your child are firm pressure and slow movement.

Activities

Movement, touch and pressure

- Jump on a trampoline or tractor inner tube. Approximately one eighth fill the inner tube with water to stabilise it; your child can jump, hop, stand, walk around, crawl around or bounce around it on his bottom. If your child is small, hold his hands as he jumps. If it is not sufficiently steady, put your foot under the inner tube to stabilise it. Invent games: when he is walking around it, go quickly, then slowly, then change directions. As your child stands on the inner tube, he can catch and throw beanbags with a bucket, play Grip ball or hit a ball down with the rolling pin.
- Zoom or orbit around on a scooter board. Your child can hold on to a hoop or towel. If he is small, he can sit on a towel or sheepskin in a cardboard carton or foam box, which sits on the scooter board, and be pulled around. He can spin himself on the spot while lying prone on the scooter board.
- Roll along a rope line, and place a jigsaw piece in position, or quoits at one end of the line. Your child then places the pieces or quoit on the other end of the line after rolling there; he can roll with a ball between his ankles.
- Roll up in a rug on the floor (Fig A3.1) or on the grass.
- Your child sits or lies across the net or vertical or horizontal car tyre. Swing him back and forth and round and round; changing directions every 30 seconds. Your child can do this himself if he lies across the net or tyre. He can catch a ball at the same time. When he is sitting in the net, he can catch a ball or small toy animals.

Prone extension

(Lying on the tummy, face down, arching up like a banana with the arms up and out to the side, and the legs raised off the scooter board or floor.)

- Your child lies prone on a car inner tube, with her chest and hips on the tube; have her arch up and catch and throw a ball (Fig A3.2). This activity is difficult –

it can usually be done only 6–10 times but it is a good substitute for one that requires suspended equipment.

- Your child lies prone in a net or across a horizontal car tyre. Push him back and forth and have him catch animals, beanbags (in a bucket) or a ball, or hit a ball with a rolling pin. He can swing or spin himself if the equipment is positioned so that he can touch the ground.

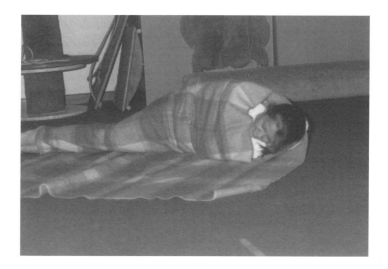

Figure A3.1: Rolling up in a rug

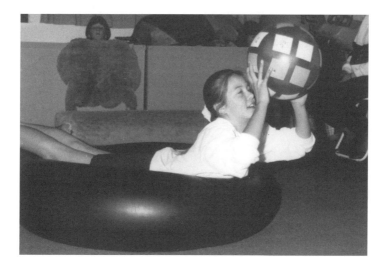

Figure A3.2: Lying prone across an inner tube and catching a ball

- Your child lies on a scooter board. Have her push off from the wall (Fig A3.3), arch up and catch a ball (Fig A3.4). Make sure that she assumes a good 'banana' posture. This activity is also hard, and your child may be able to do only 6 to 10 zooms and catches before complaining!
- Your child can do 6 to 10 arches up while he lies on the floor (e.g. watching television). Although this activity is not as effective as one that involves more movement, it works and benefits older children especially.
- Your child can carry out activities lying face down over an adult beanbag.

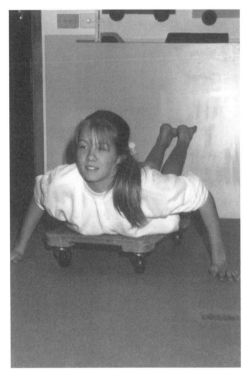

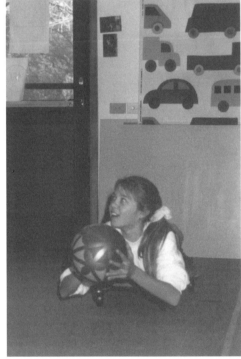

Figure A3.3: Pushing off against the wall, prone on a scooter board

Figure A3.4: Catching a ball after pushing off against the wall

Supine flexion

(Lying on the back and curling up in a ball, with the knees bent, head raised and arms up).

- Your child lies on her back on the scooter board and you hold on to her hands and whizz her back and forth between your legs (Fig A3.5). (Fathers may be able to sustain this activity longer than mothers!)

- Your child lies supine on the floor, with the hips flexed, and kicks a beachball that you throw from about waist height (Fig A3.6). This makes your child keep her head up.
- Lying on her back on the scooter board, your child pushes off from the wall with her feet and catches a ball (Fig A3.7) with her hands or feet. Stand near the wall and face your child as she zooms back.

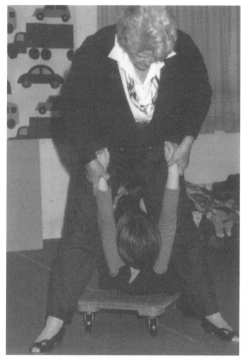

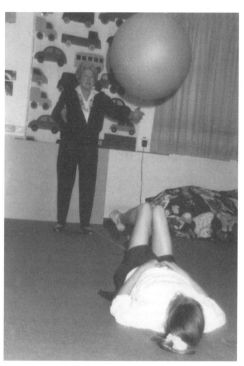

Figure A3.5: Lying supine and zooming between the parent's legs

Figure A3.6: Lying supine and kicking a beachball

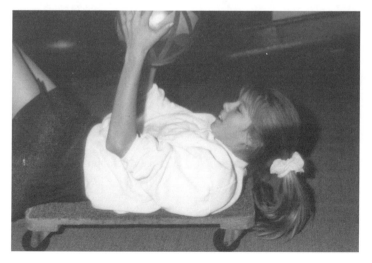

Figure A3.7: Pushing off from the wall, lying supine and catching a ball

Bilateral activities

(Both sides of body work together, so that both arms or both legs move together.)

- Your child stands on an inner tube and holds a rolling pin at both ends. He hits the ball down and back to you. You bounce the ball towards your child.
- Your child hits a suspended bag (such as an onion sack or pillow case filled with foam scraps) or small inner tube with a rolling pin (Fig A3.8). She can also hit across her body midline if she holds the rolling pin at one end with both hands and hits the suspended bag or inner tube (Fig A3.9).
- Place on the floor a length of rope, a chalk line or coloured insulation tape. Your child jumps forwards with his feet together along the line, or either side of the line, and then backwards. He holds articles, such as a soft toy animal, balloon, air-inflated empty wine cask bladder or ball, between his ankles. A modification of this acitivity is to jump between straws placed 30 cm apart, or on Twister spots or chalk circles drawn on the path outside.

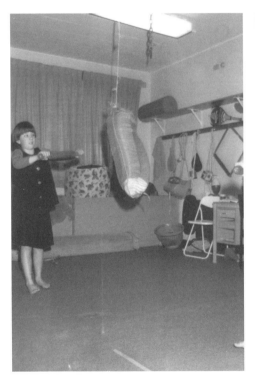

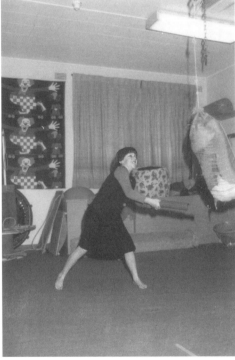

Figure A3.8: Hitting an onion sack, straight on, with a rolling pin

Figure A3.9: Hitting an onion sack across the midline with a rolling pin

Building up muscle tone

- All activities that involve jumping or activities in the movement/touch/pressure group build up muscle tone (making the tension in the muscles stronger).
- Any 'push/pull' on a joint builds up muscle tone. One example is wheelbarrowing, in which your child takes weight on his hands and you hold his legs as he 'walks' along the floor (Fig A3.10). Alternatively, have a tug o'war, or get your child to pull on a towel when he is in the net.
- Your child stands very stiffly and his sibling tries to push him over or pull him down. Then they change places.

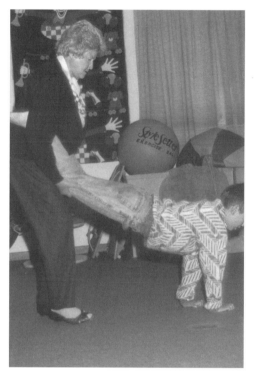

Figure A3.10: Wheelbarrowing on the hands and arms

Eye pursuits

- All eye–hand co-ordination activities with a movement/touch/pressure basis are good for eye pursuits (eye movements when tracking).
- Eye-tracking, following a moving object, such as holding a ball 30 cm away (Fig A3.11) and moving it in a 'box and cross' pattern. You can use the same pattern

to give eye-tracking at teeth-cleaning time. Ask your child to follow the tooth-brush with his eyes. Using two torches, you move one torchlight while your child keeps his head in the midline and follows your torchlight's path with his own.
- Simple fine motor activities (held off your child's the lap) while bouncing to rhythm are good. Your child can bounce on a tractor inner tube or something 'springy' (like a bed) and read a book out aloud while holding it at eye level, or do a simple jigsaw or constructional toy while bouncing, or thread a sewing card.

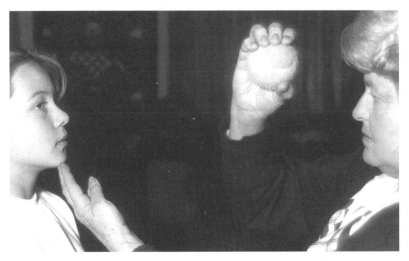

Figure A3.11: Following the movement of an object for eye pursuits

Balance

- Walk on stilt blocks or cans, forwards, backwards and cross-legged along a 'path' on the floor, or between the rungs of a ladder placed flat on the floor.
- Walk with one foot straight in front of another along a line or walk cross-legged (Fig A3.12) or backwards.
- Walk along a line or balance beam, with a book balanced on the head.
- Trampoline work, catching, walking quickly, changing directions and hitting a balloon thrown to him.
- Sibling competition: standing on one leg 'like a flamingo'.

Gross motor planning

- Bounce the ball and jump with feet together.
- Jump in spaces between small cardboard boxes placed 30 cm apart.
- Jump either side of a rope serpentine path (your child can walk along it while crossing his legs or wearing swimming flippers).
- Jump on Twister spots (forward two, back one, forward two, back one and so on).

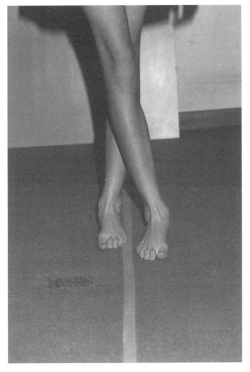

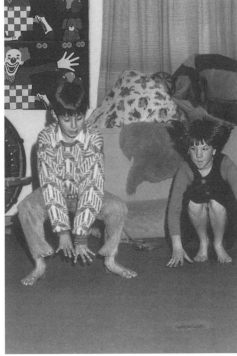

Figure A3.12: Walking cross-legged along a line

Figure A3.13: Pretending to be frogs for motor planning

- Pretend to be an animal (rabbit, duck, crab, frog (Fig A3.13), bucking donkey or kangaroo).
- Pretend to be a pirate with one eye and one leg (Fig A3.14).
- Lie on a carpet, forming numbers or letters with body (Fig A3.15).
- Play 'Simon says'.
- Jump in and out of drawn circles or hoops, with the feet together, forwards, sideways and backwards (Fig A3.16).
- Walk in unusual types of patterns (for example, use the knee of one leg and the foot of another; Fig A3.17); bend the knees slightly (Fig A3.18); walk like a toy soldier, with the same arm and leg moving together (rather than reciprocally, which is the normal walking pattern).
- Jump over a rope that you move slowly back and forth like a snake.
- Place a long rope on the floor so that the rope crosses itself many times. Your child walks along the rope and jumps over each crossing.
- Place your child in the crawl position on the scooter board with one arm and one leg off it pushing on the floor, and one arm and one leg on it (Fig A3.19).

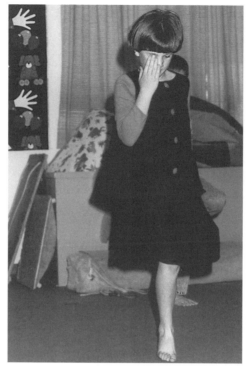

Figure A3.14: Pretending to be a pirate for motor planning

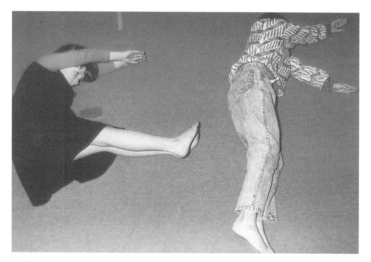

Figure A3.15: Forming letters with the body for motor planning

Gross visual space perception

- Crawl through hoops, a car inner tube or chairs.
- Crawl around chairs in a figure-of-eight pattern, first with the eyes uncovered and later with a paper bag over the head to occlude vision.

- Lie on the scooter boards and propel himself between the legs of tables or chairs – backwards, forwards, prone and supine.
- Have him crawl around cardboard cartons that you have arranged to form a maze.

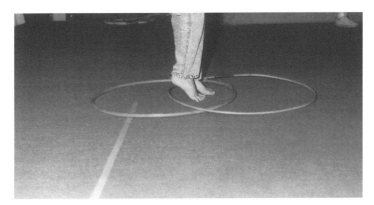

Figure A3.16: Jumping into and out of circles for motor planning

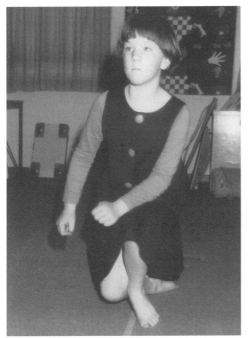

Figure A3.17: 'Walking' on one knee and one foot

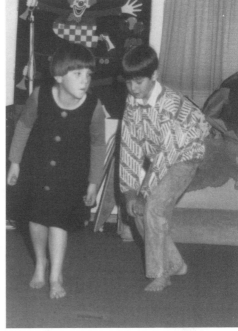

Figure A3.18: 'Walking' with the knees slightly bent

Fine motor/visual space skills

Your child should carry out fine motor skills while he is moving gently; many senses are stimulated and it is therefore more effective. You and he can sit on the tractor inner tube together while you move. Your child must have good trunk stability for him to do fine motor skills.

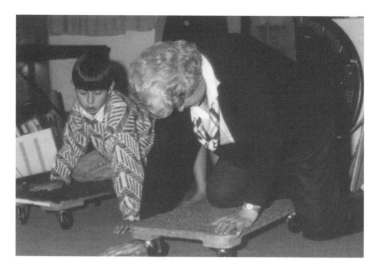

Figure A3.19: Moving along scooter board with one hand and one knee

- Cut out different shapes from coloured Playdo.
- Use dough, modelling clay or other such materials (available at art and craft supply stores). The dough can be cooked later. Make a long 'snake' and roll it into a snail, construct a face with eyes, eyebrows, nose and mouth, or make models or jewellery.
- Play with hand shape cards. Have a selection of bright yellow cards with various hand shapes drawn on them and coloured in in black. Draw curled hands; hands with one or two fingers or thumb out to the side – any variety of hand postures. Your child places his hands on these abnormal positions.
- Thread beads, macaroni, plastic tubing cut into small pieces, buttons, bottle-tops or thin strips of coloured paper rolled around a knitting needle, to make a necklace.
- Create mosaics.
- Draw and play 'boxes' or follow a maze on the white or blackboard.
- Sew around designs on cards (using old greeting cards).
- Play commercially available fine motor games, such as Lego, Duplo, peg-in-the-hole games, interlocking building blocks and constructional games.
- Weave paper strips or make paper chains.
- Make collages from strips torn out of magazines, shells, leaves, macaroni, string and coloured wool.
- Play dot-to-dot and line games.
- Make articles from matchsticks or lolly sticks.

Fine visual space perception activities

- Match picture cards, numbers or pictures on overturned playing cards ('memory').
- Play Chinese Checkers whereby your child copies a design by moving little coloured balls into holes.

- Copy a design from coloured blocks, already constructed. Vary the complexity.
- Copy letters, numbers or a design in wet sand.

Learning

- Your child bounces gently on a trampoline, mini-trampoline (or jogger), tractor inner tube or bed, or bends and straightens his knees, while she reads aloud, learns tables or words from the spelling list (Fig A3.20). This activity can help improve your child's memory for them. The input from many of the senses facilitates effective learning.
- Your child can do some writing practice with a Stetrogrip (or similar special pen grip). He can pinch pegs to strengthen his fingers and improve his grip for his pen. If your child writes very heavily in his book, he can lessen this pressure by writing on paper placed on a piece of carpet: he will pierce the paper if he does not write more lightly. He could also try doing some of his homework lying prone if he has lower muscle tone.

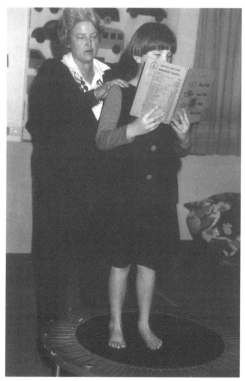

Figure A3.20: Bouncing gently on a mini-trampoline while learning

Calming

Calm your child at the conclusion of the session so that he finishes feeling relaxed. Some children need to be calmed because they are very active. If your child is very active, introduce fine motor and fine visual space activities before or during the calming activities. Fine motor activities are all-absorbing and calming.

- Slow movement and deep pressure. Hold your child in your lap and gently rock him while he watches something intriguing (a sand window, bubble novelties or egg-timers – preferably with different lengths of time) or carries out a quiet activity.
- Lie your child on the floor. Stroke right down either side of his vertebral column with your index and middle fingers; vibrate over his back or stroke him with your hands or tactile objects (a brush, sheepskin piece, feather duster or paint brush). Remember that the activity should be pleasant and relaxing for the child, otherwise it may elicit a tactually defensive response.
- Lie your child on a sheepskin on the floor and roll a large therapy ball firmly over him. Lean heavily on the ball as you roll it.

Bedwetting

Ensure that your child is calm before he goes to bed. If necessary, use the calming techniques. Place a beach towel, large toy or 'bolster' alongside him. You can make a bolster by wrapping two pillows in a beach towel. Pin the towel first to check whether it is successful and then sew it. Restrict the child's late-evening drinking. Eliminate all milk products and concentrated fruit juice from the child's diet for two weeks. Some children are intolerant of these, and this intolerance may contribute to their bedwetting. Occasionally, a child is sensitive to the chemicals in water, so it is not the amount of water consumed but the chemicals *in* the water that are causing the problem.

Most children achieve bladder control by the age of four years. Children who continue to wet the bed beyond this age, for no apparent medical reason (a check with the local doctor being essential), may be helped by the interventions as described above.

Activities for children whose parents cannot participate in the home programme

- Lie across a net or vertical car tyre and swing or spin yourself.
- Jump on the trampoline, mini-trampoline (or jogger) or tractor inner tube.
- Spin or zoom yourself on the scooter board on the floor.
- Jog on the spot, moving your arms and legs reciprocally. You can march on the spot in between your homework activities.
- Learn your spelling and times tables and practise your reading while you bounce gently to a rhythmical pattern on a trampoline/tractor inner tube, jogger or springy bed. It really helps.
- Have fun!

Appendix 4
Equipment

Sources for items of equipment that are marked by * are listed at the end of the appendix.

You will need one of each item unless stated otherwise.

Animals–small, soft, furry (10)
Balance boards (variety)
Balance bubble
Balls (2) - light/inflatable
Barrel
Basket (shoes, etc.)
Beanbag – adult
Beanbags – small (12)
Bilateral cups
Blanket – light, double-bed size
Board – black or white
Bolster – bedwetting
Bolster swing
Broom handles (2)
Calming objects (variety)
Cardboard bricks (8)
Cardboard mats (variety)
Chinese Checkers
Chinese hat/Big Top
Clown – inflatable
Constructional games (variety)
Dual swing
Exercise putty
Fine motor planning games (variety)
Fine visual space games (variety)
Four-rope platform swing
Four-rope horizontal car tyre
Frisbee

Gigantos hard plastic saucer
Hard plastic ball/therapy ball (Gigantos)
Hoops – cane or plastic (4)
Inner tube barrel
Insulation tape (variety of colours)
'J' hooks – for same number of suspended chains
'Little Tykes' enclosed, small child's swing
Log bolster
Mini-trampolines/joggers (2)
Nets (3 – 1 regular, 1 lined with sheepskin, 1 large)
Parachute
Pillow – large, foam
Plastic toy box – like a milk crate
Postrotary nystagmus board
Quoits (2 sets)
Ramp
Rolling pins (2)
Rope
Round rubber discs (8)
Rubber mat – bathroom, tactile, 'time out'
Sand buckets (2)
Scooter boards (2)
Sheepskins (2)
Shockrope-aeroplane horse
Sink plungers (2–4)

Sit'n'spin	Tennis balls (2)
Skimmer rings	Tether ball (suspended on a string)
Southpaw Flexion T Bar	Therapy balls (variety of sizes)
Southpaw safety rotational device and height adjuster	Towel tunnel
Southpaw therapy rope with eye splice	Towels – regular size (2)
Space Hopper	Tractor inner tube
Speedball	Truck inner tube
Spider ball	T-stools – of different heights (2)
Stetrogrips/pen grips	Tunnel (spiral, wire)
Stickball (1 set)	Twister game
Stilt blocks (2 pairs)	Vertical car tyre
Swimming flippers (2 pairs)	Vibrator
Swivels	Wall hanging
Tactile objects (variety)	'Witches' hats' (6)
Telephone cable rollers (2)	Wooden box-large

Treatment room

The more space you have available the better, but a room that is approximately 15.0 m × 10.0 m is functional. The room should ideally have good-quality vinyl floor covering with a heavy, removable carpet (3.0 m × 2.5 m) that can be placed where it is required. A carpeted working surface causes too much resistance to the equipment while it is being used. As much equipment as possible should be covered with soft carpet; bathroom carpet is good.

Have the maintenance specialist attach at least two strong chains to the ceiling approximately 3.9 m apart and ensure that these are checked regularly by the maintenance staff for safety. The suspended chain, together with the 'J' hook, should be long enough for you to be able to place the equipment onto the hook with ease. To the free end of each chain, attach a large (approximately 120 mm) 'J' hook with a shackle (Fig A4.1). I recommend 'J' hooks* because they can be hooked easily into the rope loops attached to each item of equipment that needs to be suspended (Fig A4.2). Each item is sufficiently heavy to stay in position. A third hook, more centrally placed in the room (to allow for a child in suspended equipment to be orbited with safety), needs to have a swivel D (Fig A4.1) so that equipment used in rotary movement spins easily and does not tangle. Allowance has to be made for the child to swing out and not hit other equipment. Attach large coat hooks to the wall at 1 metre intervals for hanging up equipment that is not in use.

Animals or puppets – soft, small and furry.

Balance boards * with curved bases (Fig A4.3); a hub cap base; five upholstery springs between two boards (have two of these with different strengths in the upholstery springs) (Fig A4.4). Cover all the boards with carpet.

Balance bubble, made of fibreglass (Fig A4.5). The base is a half circle and the top is flat and covered with soft carpet. I had one especially made for me; although it was expensive, it has been put to good use.

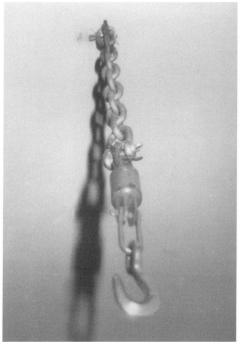

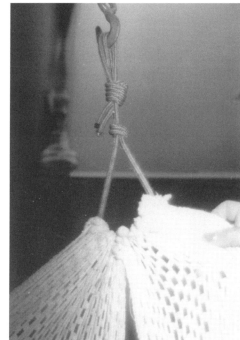

Figure A4.1: A 'J' hook

Figure A4.2: A 'J' hook with a threaded net suspended on it

Balls *. Select inflatable, hard, rubber or plastic balls that bounce well on *your* floor.

Barrel *. Line a plastic barrel with carpet. The carpet must cover the outer edge because some plastic barrels have sharp rims. An alternative barrel can be made from a large chemical container (Figs A4.6 and A4.7).

Basket for shoes, jumpers, hats, objects in pockets, etc. so that articles are never left behind nor strewn around the room.

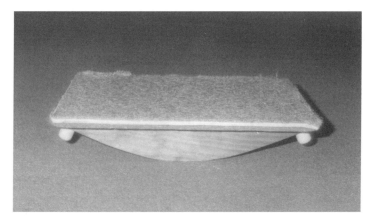

Figure A4.3: Balance board with a curved base

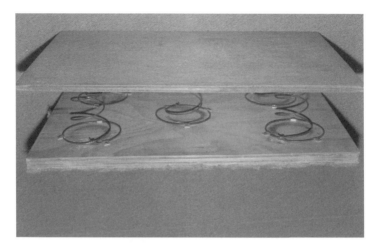

Figure A4.4: Balance board with upholstery springs

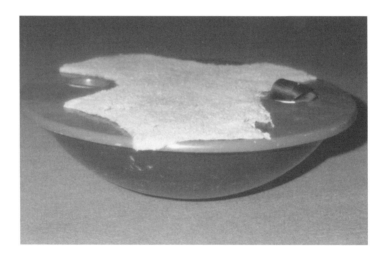

Figure A4.5: Balance bubble

Beanbags. Fill cloth bags (30 mm × 30 mm) with rice, beans, split peas or sand, and sew up the tops.

Beanbag – large, adult.

Bilateral cups made from the top halves of two 2 litre detergent bottles. Cut these in half longitudinally and join them by tape down and around the centre (Figs A4.8 and A4.9).

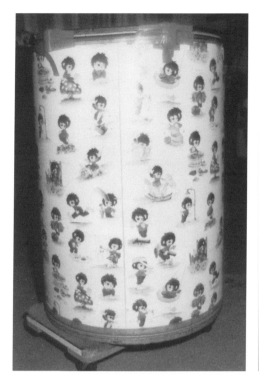 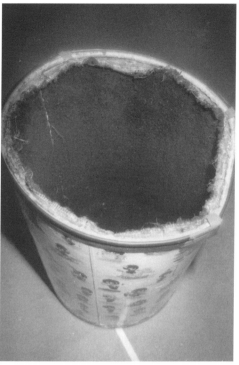

Figure A4.6: Barrel   **Figure A4.7:** Barrel, showing the inside lined with carpet

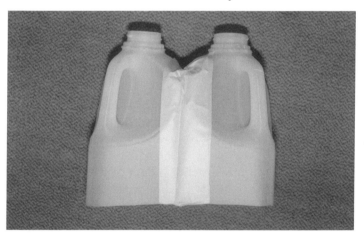

Figure A4.8: Bilateral cups

Blanket. Have a light, double-bed-size blanket for rolling in or swinging a small child in.

Board – black or white, with chalk or pens.

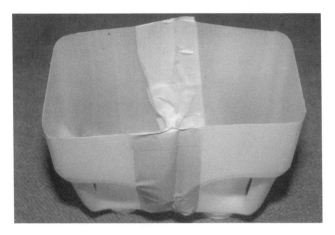

Figure A4.9: Bilateral cups, showing the inside

Bolster for treating bedwetting, to demonstrate to parents how it is made. Oversew two adjacent sides of a large (or beach) towel and put two pillows inside. If the bolster proves successful, the mother can sew up the towel more firmly by machine.

Bolster swing *. A hollow box (1.8 m × 0.15 m × 0.15 m): *a solid block of wood is too heavy to lift up and down.* Cover the box with foam (100 mm thick) and then with soft bathroom carpet. Attach two eyebolts to each end of the covered box. (The use of only one eyebolt at each end makes the swing unstable.) Attach rope to both eyebolts at each end, the rope coming up to a peak and being knotted. (see Figs 3.4 and 3.5 pp 41, 42) It is finally looped at the top to attach it to the 'J' hook at the required height.

Broom handles – two, with a crutch tip or suction cups on the end.

Calming objects. The vibrator is essential. Use sheepskin, a large therapy ball, a net, a deflated ball, a Gigantos saucer and 'intriguing' objects (such as a sand window, bubble novelties and egg-timers – preferably with different lengths of time).

Cardboard bricks or wooden blocks. Reinforce the central portion of strong boxes (for small children to walk on) and paint them or cover them with attractive adhesive covering (Fig A4.10). Wooden blacks can be the same size as a brick (230mm × 110 mm × 75mm)

Cardboard mats bearing letters or pictures. Cut cardboard (0.8 m × 2 m) and draw pictures or letters on the pieces. When the children are swinging on the horizontal tyre, they throw beanbags onto the pictures or letters and name or describe these.

Chinese Checkers.

Chinese hat/Big Top.

Clown – inflatable, of durable vinyl or plastic as children give it 'hard' wear.

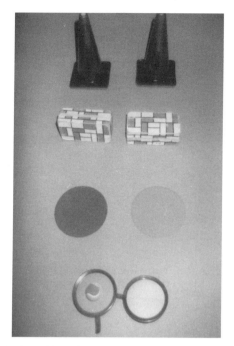

Figure A4.10: 'Witches' hat', cardboard bricks, rubber discs and stick or Grip ball

Constructional games, for example Lego, Duplo and Meccano.

Dual swing *. The swing is made of plaited nylon rope with webbing for the loops (Fig A4.11). You must reinforce the loops with soft lambswool (Fig A4.12) otherwise it hurts the child's legs.

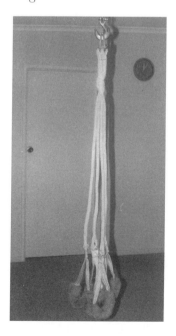

Figure A4.11: Dual swing

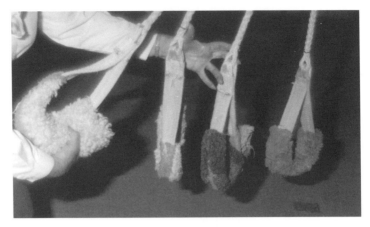

Figure A4.12: Dual swing loops reinforced with soft lambswool

Another type can be made from the largest size car or truck inner tube (Fig A4.13) and is very similar in function to the rope dual swing. Clean the tube both inside and out. Cut across the inner tube 100 mm at the top and 150 mm at the bottom, leaving the top and bottom intact (achieving a triangular shape with a flat apex). Cut four of these. Take four pieces of plastic hosing (100 mm long × 20 mm diameter) and place one piece under each of the top portions of the inner tube dual swing (Fig A4.14). Thread the rope through the hosing at the top of the inner tube and tie it in a knot on itself. Do this with each end of the rope. Tie knots in the middle of the rope for suspension. Be careful to keep the lengths of rope even, so that the child's legs will lie evenly when he is in the swing.

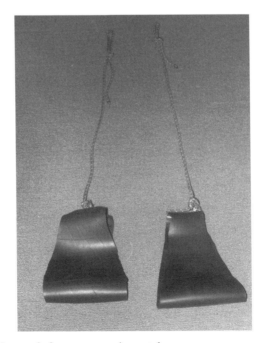

Figure A4.13: Dual swing made from a tractor inner tube

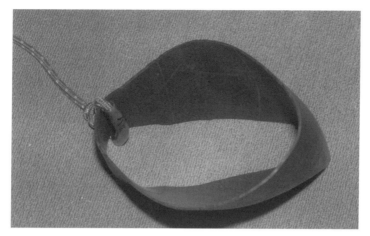

Figure A4.14: Dual swing rope threading through plastic tubing

Exercise putty

Fine motor planning/fine visual space perception activities

Four-rope horizontal car tyre. A car tyre suspended by four ropes (Fig A4.17). Drill four holes the size of a large screw-eye shank, spaced evenly apart on one side of the tyre. Insert a screw-eye in each hole and fasten it securely with a nut. Attach one end of a length of rope in two of the four screw-eye holes and then bring the other end down to the other two screw-eye holes. Tie the ropes together at the top, making a loop. This loop slips easily over the suspended 'J' hook. Have a sheepskin available to place over the edge of the tyre, if the child lies across it or inside it and leans against it to swing himself. The sheepskin lessens the hardness of the rubber.

Four-rope platform swing *. A carpeted wooden platform (0.6 m × 0.6 m) with holes drilled 250 mm in from the ends (Fig A4.15). The ropes are the length required according to the distance of the hooks from the ceiling. Two pieces of shock-rope * (3 m long) form an inverted 'U' piece, and the ends go into each hole in the base, being knotted underneath (Fig A4.16). A loop of rope is attached to the centre of the shock-rope and a knot formed, which is attached to the 'J' hook.

Frisbee

Gigantos hard plastic saucer

Hard plastic ball (Gigantos) Fig A4.18

Hoops *– cane or plastic, 90 mm × 15 mm. Bind two hoops together with insulating tape for added strength and to maintain their shape.

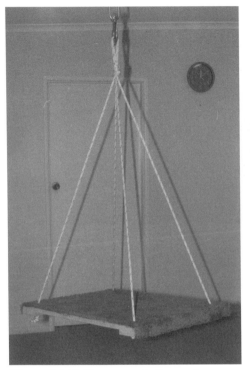

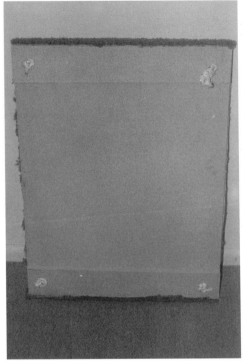

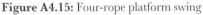

Figure A4.15: Four-rope platform swing

Figure A4.16: Four-rope platform swing with the rope knotted underneath

Inner tube 'barrel'. A cloth-covered 'barrel' made from five car inner tubes (Fig A4.19). Select five airtight, inflated tubes. Inflate the tubes and leave them up for a week to make sure that they do not leak before proceeding with the construction. Alternatively, the local garage will do this for you, as well as repairing any leaky tubes. Press down the valve stems and bind them with insulation tape, align the valve stems before you join them all together. Apply contact gel adhesive to the uppermost sides of two inner tubes. Leave this to dry until tacky and then apply a second coat. When that is also dry and tacky, join two tubes together, making sure that the valves are aligned. Repeat the procedure until all five tubes have been joined together. Reinforce the joints by binding all the tubes together with four equidistant lengths of blind cord (or similar) (Fig A4.20).

Cover the tubes with prefabricated tubular stretchy cloth, or join a piece of similar cloth along the side. Understitch each end of the cloth, being particular about the length so that it just goes over the ends of the inner tubes but does not cover the hole nor slip off. Thread elastic through the understitched opening and tie it up tightly to keep the cloth on the tubes. Sew a towelling tube inside or place a sheepskin on the valves, to increase the tactile experience. The child can roll in this 'barrel' on the floor, or you can suspend the barrel with a rope that passes through the tubes and is knotted on the outside. Tie a loop at the free end to attach the rope to a hook.

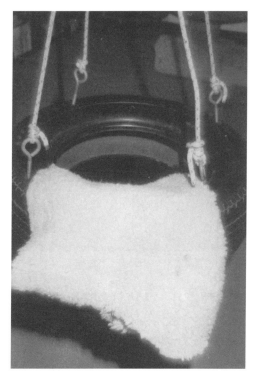

Figure A4.17: Four-rope horizontal car tyre

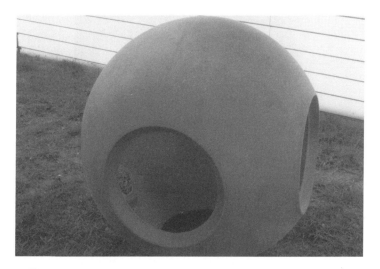

Figure A4.18: Therapy ball

Insulation tape. Have a variety of colours. Create lines on the floor – straight, in a maze, curved – using insulation tape, or paint if routine floor cleaning destroys the tape.

'J' hooks *. Hooks from which to hang equipment (see Figs A4.1, A4.2).

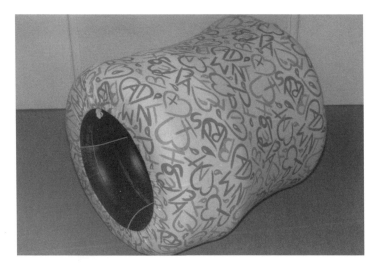

Figure A4.19: Inner tube barrel

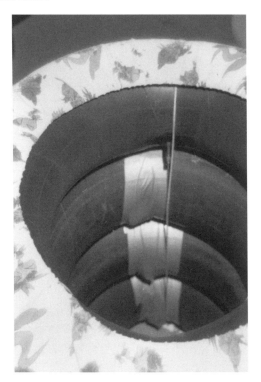

Figure A4.20: Inner tube barrel, showing the inside

'Little Tykes' swing *. A small, safe and supporting swing that can be used with babies, toddlers and pre-schoolers

Log bolster *. An inflatable vinyl cylinder (1.8 m × 0.6 m) (Fig A4.21), with a bladder inside. It laces at one end after the bladder is inflated by 'blowing out' of a vacuum cleaner.

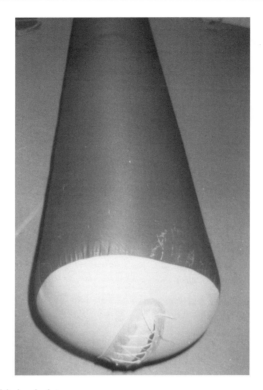

Figure A4.21: Inflatable log bolster

Mini-trampoline/joggers * (Fig A4.22).

Nets *. 2 metres per net are required. Cut and stitch each end to allow rope to be threaded through (see Fig A4.2). Fold it in half. Construct two nets from the soft material used for bouncinets. One should have the sitting area lined with a piece of sheepskin for smaller children (Fig A4.23) and another should have one edge that is bound with soft material, so that the child's armpits are not hurt (Fig A4.24). Thread, mountain-climbing rope (soft nylon non-stretch rope) through the top. Attach two 0.4 m lengths of blind cord, tied at the middle of the cord, to each side of the net to tie the child in. A larger net *, usually used for bigger and older children, can be lined with a woollen Greek floor rug (0.9 m × 1.5 m).

Parachute *.

Pillow – large foam. Use two double-bed sheets, sewn nearly completely round and stuffed to capacity with large pieces of foam. Have an outside cover of strong, durable, attractive material for protection. This can be made even more interesting and stimulating if materials of a variety of textures are applied to the covering.

Plastic toy box – like a milk crate, with a soft 'tactile' rubber mat over it, it can be used for children to have as a step up to the ramp or as the 'time out' chair.

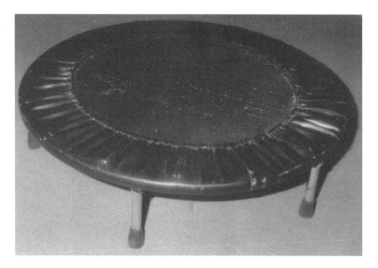

Figure A4.22: Mini-trampoline/jogger

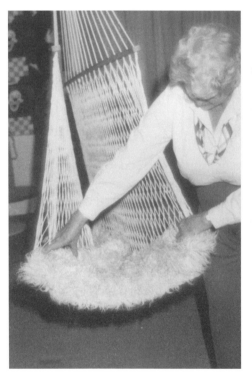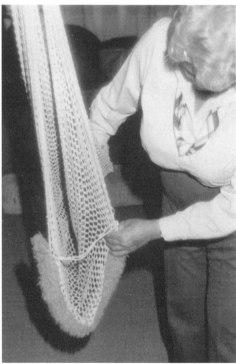

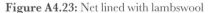

Figure A4.23: Net lined with lambswool   **Figure A4.24:** Net padded on one side

Postrotary nystagmus board *– for testing and for putting equipment on. A ballbearing swivel device can be bolted to two pieces of five-ply wood. The top piece is approximately 400 mm × 400 mm and is covered with carpet (Fig A4.25). The underneath piece is smaller, hexagonal in shape and is approximately 300 mm × 300 mm in diameter (Fig A4.26).

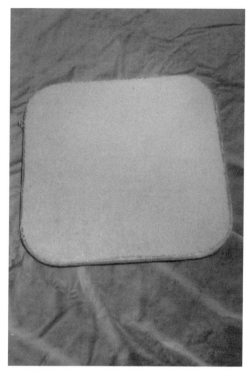

Figure A4.25: Postrotary nystagmus board – top

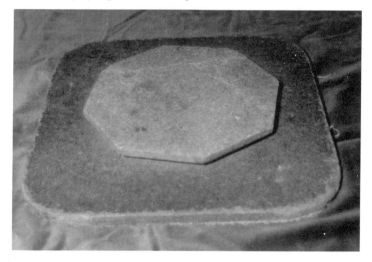

Figure A4.26: Postrotary nystagmus board – underneath

Quoits – 2 sets

Ramp (Fig A4.27). A wooden plank (3.9 m × 0.9 m) with a 5 cm ledge around the top and down the sides. The 'launching' platform at the top is square (0.9 m × 0.9 m). The romp platform is raised to a height of 0.8 m by metal legs. The ramp should slope from the edge of the platform at the top, to the floor, so that the scooter board glides off smoothly. The bottom end can be reinforced with a metal strip or solid wood, the important point being that the bottom edge is flush with the floor so that the scooter board rides off smoothly. If the room is small, use a smaller ramp or one that can be taken apart for storage. Do not carpet the ramp because carpet slows the scooter board.

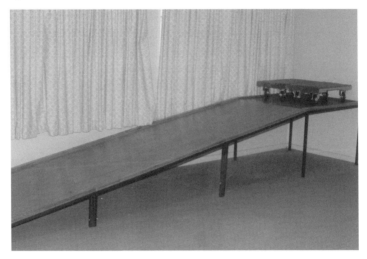

Figure A4.27: Ramp

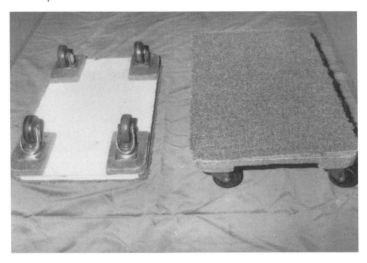

Figure A4.28: Scooter boards

Rolling pins (2). Cover the handles of each rolling pin with carpet.

Rope. Have 3 m for motor planning activities.

Round rubber discs *. Cut discs (250 mm diameter × 3 mm thick) that will lie flat and be heavy enough not to curl at the edges (see Fig A4.10). Thick matting can be used.

Rubber mat. Have a bathroom mat that has fine, soft, tiny rubber, finger-like projections on the top.

Sand buckets or the top halves of detergent bottles (held by the handles).

Scooter boards *. Acquire a solid timber board large enough for a big teenager and supportive enough for a small child. It is a carpeted wooden board (0.45 m × 0.31 m × 20 mm thick) to which castors are affixed. Use top-quality castors that have a base plate (*NOT* the peg type). If you are using ball castors, place them in pairs 50 mm in from the edges so that both right-sided castors are on the same side, opposite both left-sided castors. The top-quality wheel type that runs smoothly seems to be far more durable (Fig A4.28). It is necessary to have two scooter boards.

Sheepskins (2) – with long fibre.

Shock-rope horse *. Have a prefabricated swing seat with metal ends; thread a piece of aeroplane shock-rope through the ends and double it. Knot the ends to give you the correct height of the seat from the floor (it may be your hip height, as it sinks down when you and/or the child is sitting on it). Before sitting on it, place a sheepskin on the seat (Fig A4.29).

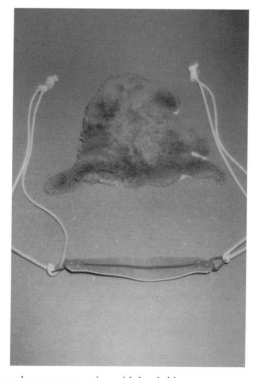

Figure A4.29: Shock-rope horse construction with lambskin

Sink plungers (2–4).

Sit'n'spin * (Fig A4.30). The seat is on ball-bearing castors. The child sits on the seat cross-legged around the central peg and holds onto the top wheel as he turns himself around.

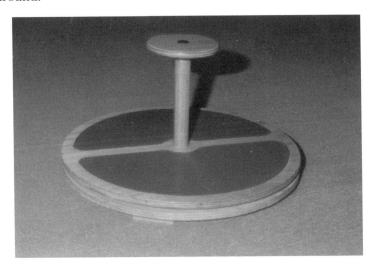

Figure A4.30: Sit'n'spin

Skimmer rings

Southpaw flexion T-bar *. A circular base with a large central peg. To make one, cut a circular plywood plate (0.76 m diameter × 20 mm thick) for the base. Cover the base with carpet. The central support is a metal plumbing pipe (plus flange) and is 1.35 m long and 30 mm in diameter. This pipe is welded to a 120 mm square plate under the base of the swing. This prevents the base coming off the central portion after extensive use with heavy children sitting or standing on it. A loop for suspension is welded on top of the pipe. A rope (about 2 m in length) is knotted underneath through a hole 30 mm in from the edge. This enables you to pull and spin the flexor swing. Wrap foam (at least 120 mm thick) around the central peg and cover this with plastic and then carpet (the plastic enabling the pre-sewn carpet to slip easily over the central peg). Cover the top with carpet.

Southpaw safety rotational device and height adjuster *

Southpaw therapy rope with eye splice.

Space hopper * (Fig A4.31).

Speed ball *. Use non-friction fine cord and shorten the cord to approximately 4 m.

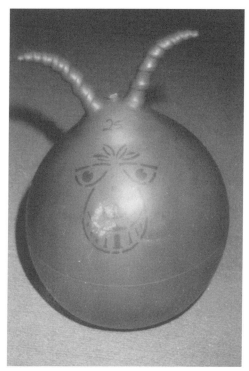

Figure A4.31: Space hopper

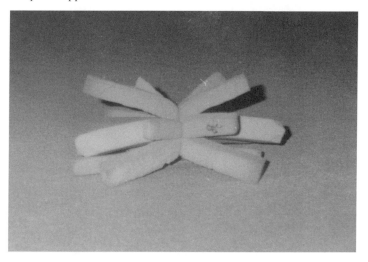

Figure A4.32: Spider ball

Spider ball (Fig A4.32) made from eight pieces of foam (300 mm × 40 mm × 40 mm). Tie all eight pieces tightly together in the centre with string. This then opens out like a pompom. It is easy for unco-ordinated children to catch or when they are moving quite considerably with an activity.

Stetrogrips or pen grips *. For writing practice.

Stick- or Grip ball *.

Stilt blocks *– bought or made, 100 mm cubed, covered with carpet. The length of rope goes through the long hole under the top, about 20 mm down. Have two pairs, one with ropes of 500 mm and one with ropes of 650 mm (for different-sized children).

Swimming flippers.

Swivel *– purchased from the named supplier is preferable, or use an adequate substitute, e.g. two nautical swivels, one attached to the ceiling hook and one attached above the 'J' hook. This allows for improved rotation of equipment.

T-stools (2), 280 mm × 250 mm, with a central peg (230 or 280 mm high). Cover the top with carpet (Fig A4.33).

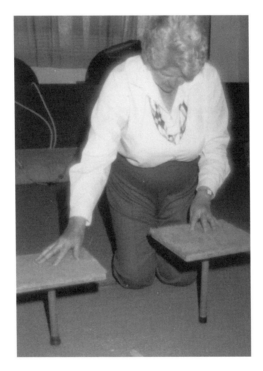

Figure A4.33: T-stools

Tactile objects – feather, woollen or cotton duster, crumb brush, soft hair brush, pot scourer, small piece of sheepskin, paint brush, make-up brush and wooden roller (Fig A4.34).

Telephone cable rollers. Two circular pieces of wood joined by a large central hub. Obtain two cable rollers (0.5 m in diameter). Attach four castors to one roller

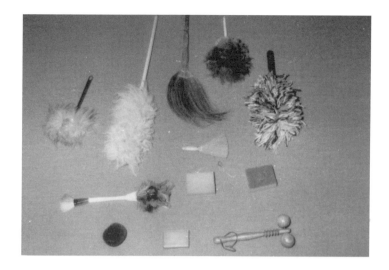

Figure A4.34: Tactile objects

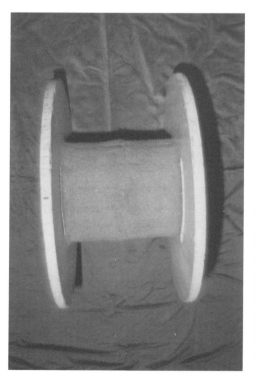

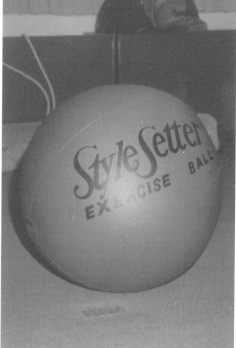

Figure A4.35: Telephone cable roller   **Figure A4.36:** Therapy ball

and tie one end of a 3 m rope to the inside of the roller (to allow for 'winding up'). Cover the top edge of the roller with carpet and attach two handles, one either side at the edge. To the hub of another reel, attach carpet (Fig A4.35) so that it can be turned on its side and walked on.

Tennis balls (2).

Tether ball (suspended).

Therapy balls *– inflatable, all sizes. The 120 cm ball (Figs A4.36, A4.18) lasts considerably longer if a vinyl covering is made for it.

Towels – regular size (2).

Towel tunnel. Sew up one side of a large towel or candlewick bedspread, or join both sides of two large beach towels. Leave the top and bottom ends free.

Tractor inner tube (Fig A4.37). Fill a tube with 2–4 litres of water to stabilise it. (Do not overfill the tube because you may not be able to manoeuvre it easily.) If the tube is particularly large or if it is not possible to fill it with water, you can still stabilise it by putting your foot underneath it while you are holding the child's hands as he jumps (see Fig 3.23 p. 50).

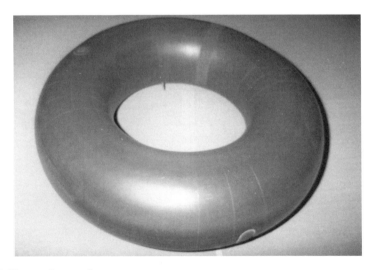

Fig A4.37: Tractor inner tube

Truck inner tube *. Inflate the inner tube well. Tie a piece of rope around it and loop it for suspending from the 'J' hook. Have another piece of rope with a loop in the middle, for suspension, and a hand piece at either end. This is made by having 100 mm of plastic tubing (20 mm in diameter) on the hand pieces, through which the rope is threaded forming a triangular handle (see Figs 3.36, 3.37, p. 56).

Tunnel *. A spiral, wire tunnel. Place a strip of carpet on the 'floor' of the tunnel (Fig A4.38).

Twister game.

Vertical car tyre, suspended vertically by one rope. Drill a hole on the outer rim of the tyre, using the same methods with the screw-eye and rope as for the four-rope car tyre. Attach a single length of rope and loop it at the top. Tie a small piece of sheepskin or thick towelling in place across the bottom of the tyre (Fig A4.39): it is too hard without some cushioning.

Vibrator *–cordless (the type that operates with a rechargeable battery) (Fig A4. 40).

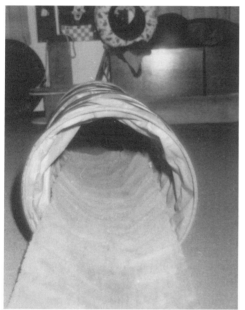 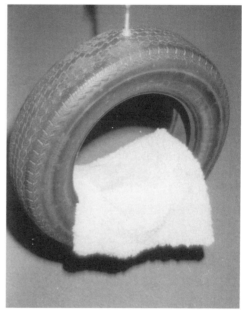

Figure A4.38: Tunnel   **Figure A4.39:** Vertical car tyre

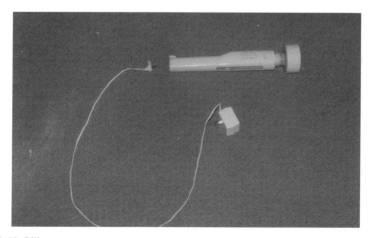

Figure A4.40: Vibrator

Wall hanging that is exciting and colourful for the children and useful for discussion of the objects on it. It can also be used as a target in throwing games.

Wooden box – large, filled with plastic coloured balls (or foam pellets). Have a large wooden box (2 m × 1 m × 0.7 m) made, or obtain a large appliance box, such as that from a refrigerator or washing machine (no smaller). Cut the box down so that the child can get in and out easily. Fill the box with coloured plastic balls or foam pellets. Balls are more expensive but much better.

Sources of equipment

Mike Ayres & Co Ltd
Vanguard Trading Estate
Britannia Road
Chesterfield
Derbyshire S40 2TZ
(+ Early Learning Centre)

James Galt & Co Ltd
Brookfield Road
Cheadle
Cheshire SK8 2PN

Hestair Hope
St Philips Drive
Royton
Oldham
Lancs OL2 6AG

Kirton Design
Bungay Road
Hempnall
Norwich NR15 2NG

Nottingham Rehab
Ludlow Hill Road
West Bridgeford
Nottingham N62 6HD

Preston Rehab Products
9–10 Standard Way
Fareham Industrial Estate
Fareham, Hants.

Hurley Aids.
123 Belmont Road,
Alexandria, NSW, 2015.
Australia,
Ph +61.2.9519 2438

Kangaroo Trading (Holdings) Pty Ltd,
P.O. Box 1055,
Brookvale, NSW, 2100,
Australia,
Ph +61.2.9938 2266
Fax +61.2.9905 2370

Modern Teaching Aids
P.O. Box 608
Brookvale, NSW, 2100, Australia
Ph + 61.2.9939 2355
Fax +61.2.9938 4082

Educational Experiences,
P.O. Box 860,
Newcastle, NSW, 2300,
Australia,
Ph +61.2.9939 2355
Fax +61.2.4942 1991

Relpar Pty Ltd,
48 Sydenham Road,
Marrickville,
N.S.W. 2044,
Australia,
Ph +61.2.9519 2943
Fax +61.2.9519 2877

Rifton
Robertsbridge
East Sussex TN32 5DR

Rompa
Goyt Side Road
Chesterfield S40 2PH
(agents for Southpaw Equipment)

Winslow Press
Telford Road
Bicester
Oxon OX6 OTS

*Equipment marked with ***

Balance boards – Rifton

Balls – Rompa

Barrel – Plastic barrel from Early Learning Centres

Bolster swing – Rompa

Dual swing – Rompa

Four-rope platform swing – Rompa

Gigantos ball and saucer – Galt

Hoops – Mike Ayres & Co Ltd and Nottingham Rehab

'J' hooks – Garages and hardware shops

'Little Tykes' Swing – Educational Experiences, Modern Teaching Aids, Kangaroo Trading, Australia

Log bolster – Similar inflatable cylinders from Rompa

Mini-trampoline – Mike Ayres & Co Ltd and Nottingham Rehab

Net hammocks – regular – Rompa

Net hammock – large – Rompa

Parachute – Mike Ayres & Co Ltd and Rompa

Postrotary nystagmus board – Western Psychological Services. Alternatively, a ball-bearing swivel device can be obtained from Hurley Aids.

Ramp

Round rubber discs – Dycem matting from Relpar

Scooter boards – Rompa

Shock-rope – this is made up of many tiny strips of elastic and is similar to luggage strap rope. The original Rompa shock-rope (13 mm in diameter) obtainable only from America, is used on aircraft carriers and is attached to netting that allow the planes to land without breaking the net.

Sit'n'spin (Twist and Turn – Carousel) – Rompa

Southpaw Flexion T-Box – Rompa

Southpaw safety rotational device and height adjuster – Rompa

Southpaw therapy rope with eye splice – Rompa

Space hopper (Hi hopper) – Early Learning Centre

Speed ball – games shops

Stetrogrips/pen grips – Early Learning Centre/LDA

Stick or Grip ball – games shops

Stilt blocks – Modern Teaching Aids, Kangaroo Trading

Swivel (rotating device) – Rompa

Therapy balls (inflatable) – Rompa

Truck inner tube – Rompa

Tunnel (wire, sprial) – Kangaroo Trading

Vibrator – Black & Decker brand, purchased from large department stores

Assessment tests

Compiled by Catherine McDerment

Bruininks-Osteretsky Test of Motor Proficiency
Robert H Bruininks (1978)
Available from: NFER-Nelson
Purpose: To measure gross and fine motor skills

Movement Assessment Battery for Children
Compiled by Sheila E Henderson and David A Sugden (1992)
Available from: The Psychological Corporation Ltd
Purpose: To identify and evaluate movement problems in children

Developmental Test of Visual-Motor Integration
Keith E Beery (1989)
Available from: Health Publishing Company
Purpose: Assessment of visual-motor skills

Goodenough–Harris Drawing Test
Dale B Harris (1963)
Available from: The Psychological Corporation Ltd
Purpose: To acquire a non-verbal measure of mental ability through assessment of a child's drawings

Miller Assessment for Pre-schoolers
Lucy Jane Miller (1982)
Available from: The Psychological Corporation Ltd
Purpose: To identify pre-school children with mild to moderate developmental delays

Screening Test for Evaluating Pre-schoolers
Lucy J Miller (1993)
Available from: The Psychological Corporation Ltd
Purpose: To identify developmental delays in young children

Sensory Integration and Praxis Tests
Available from: Preston Rehab Products
Purpose: Assessment of Sensory Integration
(NB. Requires specialised training, and scoring can only be carried out by publishing company)

Test of Visual-Motor Skills
Morrison F Gardner (1986)
Available from: Health Publishing Company
Purpose: To assess visual-motor functioning

Test of Visual Perceptual Skills (non-motor)
Morrison F Gardner (1991)
Available from: Health Publishing Company
Purpose: To determine a child's visual-perceptual strengths and weaknesses based on non-motor visual perceptual testing

Motor Free Visual Perception Test
Ronald P Colarusso and Donald D Hammill (1972)
Available from: Academic Therapy Publications
Purpose: A test of visual perception which avoids motor involvement

Address of Suppliers:
Academic Therapy Publications
21 Commercial Boulevard
Novato
California 94947

Health Publishing Co
PO BOX 3805
San Francisco
CA 94119

LDA
Duke Street
Wisbech
Cambridgeshire
PE13 2AE

NFER-Nelson
Test Department
Darville House
2 Oxford Road East
Windsor
SL4 1DF

Psychological Corporation Ltd
Foots Cray High Street
Sidcup
Kent
DA14 5HP

Appendix 5
Food Challenge Handout

This is quite safe and can be very effective for a number of children, who can be most co-operative because they feel so much better. It is necessary for the therapist to have a good understanding of this food challenge and/or work in conjunction with the dietician. Do it positively by saying, 'We are going to try to eat differently for a while. See whether you can keep to it and I will keep you in line – see who can do it best.' If you start talking about diets, everyone is bored. Many of the changes will be only temporary. Talk about what you *can* eat.

For a younger child, it is a good idea to have a chart somewhere – for example, on the fridge – and have it divided into 14 days. Place a star on each day that he or she has been co-operative. Small rewards selected and aimed for by the child are an incentive and a positive reinforcement.

You are strongly advised to get rid of all the disallowed foods from the house because you will not then be tempted to 'give in' to the child if he is being argumentative. Taste-test first to ensure that the food is tasty and acceptable; the child will not comply if the food is not acceptable.

Foods allowed

Fruit – only peeled pears.

Vegetables – acceptable ones only, such as cabbage, celery, peeled potato, lettuce, peas, beans, carrots, beetroot, asparagus, parsnip, pumpkin, turnip, sweet potato. **No tomatoes**. It is preferable to have those vegetables which are fresh in season.

Lamb, mutton, fish – all are allowed. Tuna fish in brine or water is acceptable if the can is silver-lined rather than gold-lined (which can cause a reaction for some people). Note, however, that tuna is *very high* in amines, but it is usually fine in this food challenge. The best fish is deep sea or bream – **not packet**

fish fingers. Do not give beef or veal because it can be a problem for some who have an associated milk sensitivity. Chicken is to be avoided because of the hormones and chemicals usually used in cleaning.

White or brown rice – white rice is best for some sensitive people, but brown rice is more nutritious.

Oil or margarine – use a light Spanish olive oil for cooking, and milk-free margarine for eating or cooking.

Water – plain tap water (preferably filtered), mineral and soda water are allowed.

Try to avoid any fruit juices because they can be a problem for some children. Bedwetting is common if concentrated juices are drunk. Have a can of one of the juices for an emergency for having with the *antidote* (detailed later). Pure canned pear juice without added sugar, chemicals, flavourings or preservatives may be used. Use all juices as you would for cordial – that is, a small amount in the bottom and some water added. Taste-test. The reason for dilution is that a can of pear juice could contain the juice of several pears – how long would it take you to eat this number of pears? Your child's daily consumption of juice should be similar to the rate at which she would normally eat fresh fruit. The best way of all to having some 'legal' fruit juice is to peel a pear, put it in the blender and add a little water until it is runny. Ice blocks can be made from this or from pure pear juice.

Snacks

- Rice crackers, wholegrain rice cakes or wafers.
- Papitas (dried pumpkin seeds – obtainable from health food shops).
- Sunflower seeds, cashews or any raw, unsalted nuts except almonds or peanuts (because these can sometimes be a problem).
- Plain additive-free potato crisps (thinly sliced – preferably unsalted).

Foods to be removed for 14 days

Dairy products – all types – milk (semi-skimmed, skimmed, whole or powdered), butter, margarine (except milk-free margarine), cream, yoghurt, custard, ice-cream and cheese.

Sugar group – sugar, honey, golden syrup, concentrated sweeteners, sweets and chocolate.

Yeast including Vegemite and Marmite.

Grains – cereals, except brown or white rice, including wheat, corn, oats, barley, bran, etc. This also eliminates all breads and biscuits. Although corn contains no gluten, it needs to be tested separately.

Artificial colourings, flavourings, preservatives.

Beef – steak, mince, beef sausages and veal.

Eggs.

Coffee, tea, alcohol and cigarettes.

It has been found that the foods we constantly eat and want, and the ones we avoid – are likely to be the offenders.

Do not ask anyone to eat something that he or she does not like. There are usually reasons for any such dislike to a particular food, reasons we often do not understand.

Some meal suggestions are given below. Please feel free to add your own, keeping within the allowable foods.

Breakfast

- Whole grain rice flakes with pure pear juice.
- Bubble and squeak (heated-up vegetables left over from the night before, cooked in virgin cold-pressed olive oil or light Spanish olive oil, in the form of a pancake).
- Real fish, deep-sea fish or bream are good for making fish fingers, coated in tolerated flour (do not use packet fish fingers) and chips, cooked in light Spanish olive oil. Chips can be very thinly sliced across the 'round' of the potato and fried. This is very popular with children.
- Lamb sausages, without additives.
- Chops, cutlets or other lamb and chips.
- Additive-free tuna meatballs made with mashed potato. Bind with rice flour. Cook in light Spanish olive oil. (Note the previous comment about tuna being high in amines.)
- Mashed potato cakes, cooked in light Spanish olive oil.
- Fried grated potato (oil the skillet, put the potato in to fry and turn it when brown).
- Sheep's brains rolled in crumbs. (Use crumbed rice flakes or tolerated breadcrumbs.)
- Toast or sandwiches. The best bread to use is rice bread from a health food shop. Other grain/egg/yeast/sugar/milk-free bread, rolls and muffins are obtainable from health food shops. Toast can be covered with milk-free margarine plus tahini (sesame seeds)/cashew pastes, if desired. These pastes can be obtained from a health food shop; they are expensive but are nourishing if children like them.
  It is important to slice the bread while fresh and then freeze it immediately. It will always be fresh. Use slices when needed, and toast while frozen.

- Rice cereal (obtained from a health food shop), cooked as porridge. Put into microwave oven with a little water and cook for 90 seconds. You can add a little *natural* maple syrup, obtainable from a health food shop. Another addition can be pure pear juice, which makes it very palatable.

Lunch

- Brown rice cakes, rice crackers or wafers.
- Salad.
- Cold lamb in a sandwich of special grain etc. bread with milk-free margarine. Use frozen sliced bread, which makes excellent sandwiches. For sandwiches take the slices from the freezer, spread the margarine and add the filling while the bread is still frozen. Wrap in non-waxed lunch wrapping paper. This ensures freshness by break or lunch time. Also treat slices and pancakes this way to prevent food from being unappetising.
- Home-made hot/cold soups with stock made from meat bones (not beef or veal), with the acceptable vegetables added. These are good for winter weekends.
- Pikelets (thick, small pancakes), made from rice flour, cream of tartar and bicarbonate of soda, and mashed bananas. (Bananas are occasionally acceptable.)
- Fried rice made of brown or white rice, acceptable cold meat and vegetables.
- Cold lamb meat balls, cold lamb sausages (no preservatives), cold additive-free tuna meatballs, all left over from the previous night's dinner.

Dinner

Many normal meals are already within the foods allowed. With gravies, use rice flour or arrowroot in the meat juices for flavour and colour. See also the *Breakfast* list.

Peeled pears or ice lollies made from pure pear juice are the only desserts allowed for these two weeks.

It is best to have a rotation diet – the same foods every four days rather than every day. For a maintenance programme, refer to the four-day sample in *The Allergy Tuckerbox* recipe book, by Jenny Bennett (see Recommended reading).

Reintroduction

After 14 days, reintroduce **one food at a time**, allowing a two-day period for each new food. It is important to have a moderate serving of a food to challenge it, because this will still cause some symptoms if it is a problem. For example, with milk, a blocked or snuffly nose is common. A very large serving of milk could cause cold or influenza-like symptoms and turn to infection. This sets everyone back. A suggested challenge for milk is a moderate serving (one large glass, followed by another moderate serving in two to three hours if no reaction has occurred). Always introduce foods on their own. Watch for reactions. These could be overactivity, tearfulness, excessive fatigue, aggression, irritability, tantrums, puffiness, headache, deterioration in schoolwork, anything that you think is atypical. The changes may occur immediately, within hours or even the next day. This is the reason for a two-day test period. Everyone is different so will react differently. Parents know their families and are the best judges.

For a clearer picture, give just gluten (e.g. grains), dairy and egg a four-day break to be sure there is no reaction to these commonly eaten foods. Leave introducing wheat until last because it is the slowest to be eliminated from the child's system.

If the reintroduced food causes a reaction, withdraw it immediately and allow the person to recover before further reintroducing the next food. (This usually takes about six days.)

Each food is to be reintroduced in the similar manner until the person is back on a full diet.

If the child is longing for bread, first introduce wheat by way of plain, thin wheat biscuits which are yeast-free. If she is cleared, then make a basic loaf from:

- 2 cups of wholemeal self-raising flour
- 1 full cup of water
- 1 teaspoon of salt
- Mix the dough, place in hot oven (200–215°C) for 25–30 minutes.

Next you can buy some baker's yeast at the health food store or cake shop and make some bread to test yeast. Bread has many components, which you will discover when you read the labels. If your child is reacting, you will need to know what is causing it. The only safe way is to test it.

Antidote

If you feel relief is needed from a bad reaction or withdrawal symptoms, doctors recommend a useful formula, which is one third potassium bicarbonate (from a chemist) and two-thirds sodium bicarbonate. Take a teaspoon of this combination and add to two big glasses of water – one glass of water now, followed by a second glass of water later – *not* more than twice in 24 hours, after your child has eaten the food that causes a reaction. This is the best mixture, but just half a teaspoon of bicarbonate of soda (from a chemist) and one glass of water, followed later by another glass of water with bicarbonate of soda, often helps. Add some pure pear juice to this antidote if the child is young. If the reaction is marked, she can take Pretorius Massive Cal C powder (from a health food shop) every hour until the reaction goes. If the potassium and sodium bicarbonate are not acceptable, a sachet of Citravescent or Ural is also good. Drink this while fizzing. Either is far more palatable than the bicarbonate mixture, but use sparingly. Citravescent and Ural can be obtained from a chemist.

Experience has revealed that people with food sensitivities usually improve when potentially troublesome foods are removed from their diet over a two week period. If there is a milk intolerance, for example, the milk is being malabsorbed anyway.

Some people get withdrawal symptoms, which may be quite severe. This usually lasts only up to a maximum of four days. Children may get difficult, especially when they are sugar sensitive. They can also get tearful on occasions. **Try to persist, because the reaction is significant**. Some adults get headaches or other symptoms from giving up tea and coffee. This is important because their body is trying to say something about their health.

If the child gets ravenously hungry, let him have a lot of snacks but **do not use any sweet snacks**. He will settle down after a few weeks when he has got used to the change. Some parents find it useful to have a meal ready when the child gets home from school and a lighter snack before bedtime. See the suggested week's menu (at the end of this section) for ideas, and refer to the recipe book *The Allergy Tuckerbox* by Jenny Bennett, after the two-week trial, to expand the diet.

Beware of 'trigger' foods: one bite and the trouble starts.

Rotate your child's meals from now on. Do not keep having the same food each meal. Vary the diet or your child's body may react to the sameness. This is most important. Refer to *The Allergy Tuckerbox* by Jenny Bennett for a sample maintenance menu.

If there is no difference whatsoever from the elimination diet, continue to keep off products containing gluten (wheat and grains) because that is a substance that may take up to two months to be eliminated from the system.

It is wise to read all labels and ask. For example, casein – a common emulsifier – is a milk protein.

It could be that the child's symptoms have not disappeared despite the food challenge. Because food and environmental chemical sensitivities go together, so the signs and symptoms of environmental chemical sensitivities can be similar to those exhibited by food intolerances. Environmental chemicals are not to be confused with food chemicals, that is, artificial colours, flavours, preservatives, amines and salicylates, most of which are eliminated anyway in the food challenge. It must be realised that the environmental chemical is sometimes the problem, which is why children do not react any differently when put on the food challenge programme.

If an environmental chemical is suspected as the offender, it should be removed or the child should be removed from the offending chemical. The *antidote* to a chemical reaction is the same as that used for food reactions.

Finally, an intolerance to substances in water must not be overlooked. The use of a good-quality water filter may be the answer to the problems. Bedwetting can be caused by added chemicals in the water.

Suggested menu plan

Days 1 and 8

Breakfast: Rice cereal with pure pear juice and/or grain-free toast and milk-free margarine and/or bubble and squeak with acceptable vegetables.

Break: One packet of plain, additive-free crisps with no artificial colour or special pikelets (see above) spread with milk-free margarine.

Lunch: Acceptable vegetables (salad) and additive-free tuna sandwich (Note the comment about tuna above.) Refer to comments on keeping sandwiches fresh.

After school: Cashews, sunflower seeds. **No peanuts.** Carrot sticks.

Dinner: Roast lamb, fresh acceptable vegetables (**no tomatoes**). If gravy is desired, thicken with rice flour or arrowroot. Peeled pears or ice lollies made from pure pear juice.

Days 2 and 9

Breakfast: Rice cereal and/or grain-free toast and milk-free margarine and/or meatballs made of cold lamb.

Break: One packet of plain, additive-free crisps or special pikelets spread with milk-free margarine.

Lunch: Left-over cold lamb in a sandwich. Carrot and celery sticks.

After school: Rice crackers and/or rice cakes with milk-free margarine or cashew/tahini (sesame seed) paste.

Dinner: Lamb sausages (get the butcher to make some up for you, *without preservatives*). Fresh acceptable vegetables (**no tomatoes**).
   Meat balls, made from minced lamb, or cottage pie made from minced cold lamb from the night before, with acceptable vegetables and gravy thickened with arrowroot or rice flour. Peeled pears or a pear juice ice lolly.

Days 3 and 10

Breakfast: Rice cereal and/or grain-free toast with milk-free margarine and/or additive-free tuna cakes, fried in light Spanish oil.

Break: One packet of plain, additive-free crisps.

Lunch: Left-over cold lamb sausages/meatballs in a grain-free sandwich, with milk-free margarine.

After school: Peeled pear. Rice cake with milk-free margarine.

Dinner: Fried rice of brown rice (boiled for approximately 20 minutes and well drained) or white rice if tolerated better. Add additive-free tuna and/or a few *fresh* prawns and any acceptable vegetables (**no tomatoes**). A dob of milk-free margarine binds it.
     Fried fish (deep sea fish or bream) coated with rice flour and fried in light Spanish olive oil.

Days 4 and 11

Breakfast: Real fish fingers – deep sea fish or bream makes good fish fingers. Coat in tolerated flour. **Do not use packet fish fingers**. Have with chips cooked in light Spanish olive oil and/or potato cakes, either mashed or grated and fried in the same oil.

Break: Peeled pear.

Lunch: Additive-free tuna sandwiches, mashed with some margarine added to bind it. Carrot and celery sticks.

After school: Plain, additive-free crisps. Fresh cashews. Vegetable sticks.

Dinner: Lamb chops or cutlets with fresh acceptable vegetables (**no tomatoes**). Pure pear juice ice lolly.

Days 5 and 12

Breakfast: Rice cereal with pure pear juice and/or grain-free toast with milk-free margarine/nut paste (**not peanut butter**) and/or sliced potato chips, cooked in allowable oil.

Break: Plain, additive-free crisps.

Lunch: Left-over cold chops/cutlets or the meat sliced from these and put into sliced grain-free bread sandwich, spread with milk-free margarine. Carrot sticks.

After school: Rice crackers/cakes with milk-free margarine or cashew/tahini nut paste. Peeled pear.

Dinner: Additive-free tuna rissoles with acceptable vegetables – **no tomatoes**. Peeled pear or pure pear juice ice lolly.

Days 6 and 13

Breakfast: Rice cereal and/or grain-free bread with milk-free margarine and/or bubble and squeak cooked in light Spanish oil.

Break: One packet of plain additive-free crisps.

Lunch: Left-over additive-free tuna rissoles in grain-free sandwich and milk-free margarine. Vegetable sticks.

After school: Cashews. Peeled pears.

Dinner: Lamb sausages (ask the butcher to make some up for you with **no additives**. Acceptable vegetables (**no tomatoes**). Peeled pear or pure pear juice ice lolly.

Days 7 and 14

Breakfast: Real fish fingers, made from deep sea fish or bream are good. Coat in tolerated flour. **Do not use packet fish fingers**. Have with chips cooked in light Spanish olive oil and/or potato cakes, either mashed or grated and fried in the same oil.

Break: One packet of additive-free thin crisps.

Lunch: Left-over lamb sausages. Vegetable sticks.

After school: Special pikelets and milk-free margarine.

Dinner: Fried lamb cutlets coated in rice flour or just grilled, with acceptable vegetables – **no tomatoes**. Peeled pear or pure pear juice ice lolly.

Recommended reading

Bennett J (1987) *The Allergy Survival Kit*. Available from Jenny Bennett, 19 Fiesta Crescent, Copacabana, NSW 2251, Australia.

Bennett J (1993) *The Allergy Tuckerbox*. Recipes for people with food sensitivities. Available from Jenny Bennett, 19 Fiesta Crescent, Copacabana, NSW 2251, Australia.

Hanssen M (1989) *The New Additive Code Breaker*. Lothian. Reserved for Australia by Betty Norris, Melbourne.

Mackarness R (1977) *Not All in the Mind*. London: Pan Books.

Minchin M (1986) *Food for Thought*. Melbourne: Unwin Paperbacks.

Randolph T (1981) *Allergies, Your Hidden Enemy*. New York: Wellingsborough Turnstone.

Verkerk R (1990) *Building Out Termites*. Sydney: Pluto Press. (Chemical-free control.)

Acknowledgement

This handout was compiled by Elaine B. Wilson, with additions made by Jenny Bennett. Information has been gathered over the years from parents, dieticians and nutrition specialists, working with these children.

Glossary

Aberrant behaviour: Unacceptable behaviour. Deviation from the normal and usual type of behaviour.

Basal ganglia: Structures that lie subcortically and function to control unwanted movement, enable sequencing of a task and permit slow, controlled movements. Developmentally dyspraxic children may not do these well.

Choreoathetosis: The fine uncontrolled movements of the fingers that are seen in a posturally stressed child.

Co-contraction: The simultaneous contraction of all the muscles around the joint to maintain stability.

Deep pressure: Pressure that is applied to the child's body to integrate vestibular–proprioceptive input and/or to calm the child.

Dendritic growth: Growth of the dendrites or 'branches' on the neurone (nerve cell). It is hypothesised that therapy can facilitate dendritic growth, whereby more dendrites develop on the neurone, allowing for better interconnection between neurones and thus better transmission of impulses.

Developmental dyspraxia: A dysfunction whereby there is difficulty in the actual planning and execution of the motor acts. This dysfunction has a tactile perception basis, a vestibular–proprioceptive basis or, as is more often the case, both. A child who has poor tactile perception, along with disinhibition of the higher centres could also be tactually defensive; he may have a low tactile threshold, whereby he feels very little touch and appears to overreact, or a high tactile threshold whereby he can tolerate a great deal of pain without complaint.

Differential diagnosis: The term used when selecting the correct diagnosis from several that will fit the given clinical picture.

Disinhibition: Overactivity, abnormal irritability, tactile defensiveness, distractibility, poor concentration and memory, fussiness, bedwetting and an intolerance to noise, light, smell and/or movement are all manifestations of disinhibition.

Any of these behaviours, particularly overactivity, are common reasons for parents to seek help for their children. Disinhibition can accompany hemispheral or brainstem dysfunctions. It can be closely associated with attention deficit disorder (ADD).

Exteroceptive input: Another term for input from the touch receptors.

Generalised dysfunction: This encompasses brainstem and hemispheral dysfunctions. The deficits are more extensive and more severe. A child with a generalised dysfunction often requires several blocks of therapy, ideally 6 to 12 months apart.

Gravitational insecurity: The insecurity that a child experiences in space, when his feet are off the ground and he does not have the control of his body or movement. Gravitational insecurity is associated with poor vestibular–proprioceptive processing and a poor relationship to gravity. It is seen quite commonly in children with sensory integrative dysfunction and is associated with disinhibition.

Language – expressive: The ability to express oneself verbally.

Language – receptive: The ability to understand and integrate what is being said. Speech, expressive and receptive language deficits are frequently associated with problems of sensory integration.

Left hemispheral dysfunction: Right-sided scores on formal and non-standard testing are depressed and/or lower than left-sided scores. The postural responses and brainstem integration are usually normal. Postrotary nystagmus can be hyperresponsive (often with a low tolerance to movement) or within normal limits. Speech, expressive and receptive language scores can be depressed and, rarely, behaviour problems occur. Minor problems with tactile perception can occur without developmental dyspraxia. However, deficits that are due to a left hemispheral dysfunction usually respond less favourably to sensory integrative treatment procedures.

Linear movements: Movements back and forth (bolster swing; zooming down the ramp), up and down (jumping on a tractor inner tube), and in one direction, are linear.

Multisensory input: Input that involves more than one of the seven senses being stimulated concurrently. Multisensory input facilitates improved sensory integration.

Neural inhibition: The nervous system has five times as many inhibitory fibres as facilitatory fibres. Some sensory input is inhibited by these fibres so that the brain learns to accept some information and reject other.

Neuroanatomical: A reference to the *structure* of the central nervous system.

Neurophysiological: A reference to the *function* of the central nervous system.

Nuchal ligaments: A pair of ligaments that lie at the back of the neck and extend from the occiput (back of the base of the skull) to the 7th cervical vertebra.

Occiput: A protuberance at the base of the back of the skull. Massaging the acupressure point on the occiput between the nuchal ligaments can usually reduce nausea.

Postrotary nystagmus: The reflex horizontal eye movements that occur after the body is rotated at a certain speed and then stopped suddenly. A standardised test is frequently used to assess postrotary nystagmus.

Primal reaction: An adrenaline-charged reflex that is basic to survival and is not altered by reasoning, conditioning or behaviour modification. A tactually defensive response can be a primal reaction.

Prone extension: The extension of the proximal joints (neck, shoulders, trunk and hips) that occurs when a child lies face downwards on his stomach and arches up.

Protective extension: An automatic reaction that extends the arms to provide protection when a person is falling.

Proximal stability: Stability that results from the co-contraction of the muscles around the proximal joints (neck, shoulders, trunk and hips). Proximal stability must be established before distal stability can be achieved. Proximal stability is essential for efficient mobility and fine motor control.

Regression effects: Reactions to the neural 'disorganisation' that therapy sometimes causes. Regression effects may manifest as overactivity, excessive irritability, nausea and/or headache.

Reliability: The ability of an instrument to produce the same results when applied to the same person under the same conditions. The simplest way to assess reliability is the test–retest method, in which the same instrument (or 'test') is used with the same person on two different occasions separated by a short period. Assuming that there have been no real changes in the person, the results from the two 'tests' should be the same (Cumming and Scanlon, 1994).

Interrater reliability provides evidence of the degree to which different examiners could expect to get similar scores using the test on the same individual.

Test–retest reliability 'examines whether or not a child's test scores would be constant over time if retested at a later date' (Chapter 2, p. 7).

Right hemispheral dysfunction: Left-sided scores on formal and non-standardised testing are depressed and/or lower than the right-sided scores. Postural problems, poor visual space perception and behavioural problems can be associated with a right hemispheral dysfunction. Murray (1991, p. 192) states:

> Although sensory integrative dysfunction may exist along with, and may even contribute to, cortical dysfunction, probably the actual problems these learning-disabled children experience in academic learning result from problems in cortical function.

Rotary movements: Movements that occur with activities such as orbiting (two children in the dual swing), spinning (in a net) and rolling (in a barrel).

Semicircular canals: Part of the vestibular apparatus. The vestibular apparatus and the cochlea (for hearing) lie in the inner ear.

Somatosensory information: Sensory information from the tactile receptors.

Supine flexion: The flexion of the hips, knees and neck that occurs when a child lies on his back, curls up and brings his knees towards his forehead.

Symptomatic changes: Changes (improvement or deterioration) in the symptoms for which the child was referred, for example co-ordination, school performance, speech, language or behaviour.

Tactile defensiveness: An excessive, emotional reaction to touch that registers as being unpleasant or threatening to the person. It is frequently seen in children who are referred for sensory integrative treatment procedures and is often a result of overall disinhibition.

Utricle and saccule: Part of the vestibular apparatus. The vestibular apparatus and the cochlea (for hearing) lie in the inner ear.

Validity: The degree to which an instrument measures what it is supposed to measure. The usual way of assessing validity is to compare results obtained from the selected instrument with the results obtained using another instrument that measures the same parameter (Cumming and Scanlon, 1994).

Vestibular–proprioceptive input: Input from the vestibular system and the proprioceptors in the joints, tendons and muscles.

Visual perception: The interpretation of what is seen.

References and recommended reading

Cumming R, Scanlon K (1994) *Health Promotion and Older People: A Guide for Evaluators*. (State Health Publication No HP 94 – 031.) Prepared by the Health Promotion Unit, NSW Health Department, Australia.

Murray E A (1991) Hemispheric Specialisation, in Fisher AG, Murray EA, Bundy AC (1991) *Sensory Integration: Theory and Practice*. Philadephia: Davis.

Index

Action Against Allergy 95
aggression 34
air pollution 97, 98
allergy stress 89
anger 84
anticipation 80, 83
assertiveness 34
assessment procedures 6–7
assessment rationale 7–8
assessment tests 185–6
assessment tools 8–9
asymmetrical tonic neck reflex 17, 128, 133
attention deficit disorder 3

balance 16, 18, 43, 49, 55, 57, 152
balance and trunk rotation 140
balance deficits 18
basic needs 83
bathing and cleaning 95–6
bedwetting 3, 72–3, 158, 188
behaviour 3–4, 109
    atypical 35
behaviour management 10, 35–9, 79–88
Bender-Gestalt Test 21
bilateral activities 53–4, 138–9, 150
bilateral and vestibular activity 48
birth history 102–3, 107
body language 75, 85
bolster swing 41
boundaries, physical and verbal 37
brainstem 1, 2
Bruininks–Oseretsky Test of Motor Proficiency
    3, 18–19, 101

calming 64–6, 73, 157–8
Capital Area Treatment Rating 13, 100
chemical intolerance 94–5
chemical sensitivities 10, 73, 89, 104
chemicals 94
Chinese Checkers 64, 156
clinical observation 3, 16
Clinical Observations of Motor and Postural
    Skills 17, 100
Clinical Observations protocol 16–17
Clinical Observations Test 17, 100, 127–9,
    130–4
co-contraction 128, 132
co-ordination problems 6, 20, 102–4
communication 104
concentration, poor 3, 73–4, 93, 109
conflict handling 80, 83
confrontation 84
consistency 36, 80, 83, 87
contract, parent/child 76
Coopersmith Self Esteem Inventories 24, 75,
    101
crossing the midline activity 53–4, 57, 140–1
crying 86–7

damage repair 80, 85
deep pressure 64, 72, 158
deficits, specific 4
Detroit Test of Learning Aptitude – Primary
    19, 101
Developmental Test of Visual Perception 23,
    101

Developmental Test of Visual-Motor
    Integration 23, 101, 122, 185
diadokokinesia 127, 131
Diagnosis and Remediation of Handwriting
    Problems 25, 101
disinhibition 3, 74
disorganisation 35
distractibility 3, 73, 130
documentation 7
dressing 103, 108
dual swing 42, 51
dustmite allergy 96

eating 103–4, 107
emotional growth 88
emotional skills 104, 110
environmental illness see chemical sensitivities;
    food sensitivities
equilibrium reactions 132
equipment 145, 159–60, 160–84
    safety checks 34–5
ethics 7
eye-hand co-ordination 49, 55, 57, 141–2
eye closure, independent 127, 131
eye contact 11, 76
eye movements 127, 131
eye tracking 141, 151–2

family dynamics 80–2
fatigue 93, 98
fine motor/visual space skills 63, 103, 109,
    155–6
fine visual space perception activities 64, 156–7
finger-nose touching 17
flexor swing 48
food and food additives sensitivities 10, 89, 104
    antidote 191–2
    symptoms 90–1
food challenge 10
food challenge handout 187–95
food diary 10
food elimination 92, 93, 188–90
food intolerance 92
food reintroduction 190–1
fussiness 74

glue-ear 92
Goodenough-Harris Drawing Test 18, 19
gravitational insecurity 21, 42, 74, 129, 133
gross motor planning 60–2, 152–4
gross motor skills 103, 109

gross visual space perception 62, 154–5
group therapy 87

handedness 103, 127, 130
handwriting 24, 93, 135–6
Handwriting Checklist 25, 101
Handwriting File 25
headache 34, 70
health 104
hearing 104
hearing screens 11
high tolerance to movement 70
history questionnaire 10
history taking 21
home programme 10, 40, 144–58
    activities 146–58
    equipment 145
horizontal tyre 47
hyperactivity 35, 92, 130, 143
hypertonus 77, 127, 131
hyperventilation 35
hypoactivity 92
hypoallergenic products 95

identification 9–10
immune response, abnormal 89
impulsiveness 3
Infant/Toddler Screening for Everybaby 13,
    100
Infant/Toddler Symptom Checklist 13, 100
intelligence 104
interrater reliability 7
intervention 86
Irlen syndrome 10
Irlen syndrome screening guide 117–18
irresponsibility 88
irritability 3, 34, 74

Kaufman Assessment Battery for Children 21
language, expressive and receptive 4
learning 157
learning problems 102
lifting a child safely into the net hammock 55
linear movement 41, 51, 57
linear vestibular activity 48
log bolster 57
low tolerance to movement 68–9
Luria-Nebraska Neuropsychological Battery
    21

management tools 79, 80, 82–8
masking effects, food 93
    chemicals 94
McCarron Assessment of Neuromuscular
    Development 20, 101
memory 3, 93, 104
milestones 102–3, 107
Miller Assessment of Pre-schoolers 20, 101,
    185
Miller Toddler and Infant Evaluation 14, 100
mini-trampolines 48, 57
motor deficits 17
Motor Development Checklist for Infants
    Stressed Prenatally with Maternal
    Cocaine Use 13, 14–15, 100
Motor Free Visual Perception Test 23, 101,
    122, 186
motor performance 3
motor planning ability 24, 41, 142
motor skills 103–4
    deficit 3–4
Movement Assessment Battery for Children
    20–1, 101, 185
muscle tone 16, 49, 57, 127, 130, 151

nausea 34, 69–70
NEED Centre Observation of Writing 25, 101,
    135–6
NEED Perceptual-Motor Checklist 126
net 51–3, 55
New England Educational Diagnostic Centre
    25
New England Educational Diagnostic Centre
    Screen 15, 100
non-standardised tests 16–18, 100–1

Occupational Therapy Referral Form 10, 119
Occupational Therapy Report 120–4
organic foods 93–4
overactivity 3, 10, 34, 73, 92
overstimulation 68

parachute 57–8
Parents' Questionnaire 10, 105–12
parents, anxious 79
parents, role of in therapy 39–40
Pediatric Clinical Tests of Sensory Interaction
    for Balance 18, 101
pen grip 25, 103, 125, 130, 135
picture cards 64
Piers-Harris Children's Self-concept Scale 24

play 104
positive feedback 75
positive reinforcers 35
postrotary nystagmus, hyporeactive 5
postrotary nystagmus test 122
postural adjustment 132
postural background movements 132
postural response 21
posture 134
praise 75
progress, lack of 66–7
prone extension 16, 43, 128
prone extension activities 139, 146–8
prone extension posture 17, 133
protective extension 59, 128, 132, 141
punch-bag 38

Quick Neurological Screening Test 15, 100

ramp 43–7
rapid forearm rotation 17
referral 9–10
regression effects 34, 40
reporting 12
role-play 75, 77
rotary movement 42, 47, 48, 55
rotary vestibular activity 50–1
routine 83

Schilder's arm extension posture 128; 132–3
Schilder's Arm Extension Test 17, 128
School Questionnaire 10, 113–16
scooter board 45, 55
Scototopic Sensitivity/Irlen Syndrome Screen
    14, 100, 117–18
screening 13
screening tests 100
Screening Test for Evaluating Pre-schoolers 15
seizures 35, 68
self-care 108
self-esteem tests 24
self-esteem, low 75, 76
Self-opinion Questionnaire 24
sensitivity, symptoms of 90–2
sensory defensiveness 21
sensory input 1
sensory integration 1, 2
    benefits of 4
Sensory Integration and Praxis Tests 21–2,
    101, 185
sensory integrative dysfunction 2, 3

sensory integrative activities 137–43
sensory integrative treatment procedures 2,
      137–43
sensory intolerance 3, 72
sensory perception 2
sensory registration 1
sensory stimulation 77
skills delay 6
slow motion 17, 64, 127, 131
social skills 76, 104, 110
Southern California Postrotary Nystagmus
      Test 18, 22, 68, 101
Southern California Sensory Integration Test
      19, 22, 101
speech deficits 3, 4, 75
speech therapy 75
standardised tests 18–22, 101
stroking 158
structure 36
supine flexion 16, 129, 133, 148–9
supine flexion activities 139–40, 148–9
supine flexion posture 17, 43
symmetrical tonic neck reflex 128, 133

tactile activities 138
tactile defensiveness 3, 71–2, 130
teamwork 39
tearfulness 34, 35
teasing 76–7
temper tantrums 38–9
test environment 11
Test of Sensory Functions in Infants 15, 100
Test of Visual-Motor Skills 185
Test of Visual-Perceptual Skills 23, 101, 186
test report 12
test validity/reliability 7
therapy ball 65

therapy sessions 32–4
therapy video 39
thumb-finger touching 128, 131–2
time out 37–8, 84–5
tiredness 34
tone activities 138
tongue-to-lip movements 128, 132
tonic neck reflex, asymmetrical 17
Touch Inventory for Elementary School-aged
      Children 13, 15, 100
tractor inner tube 49
treatment objectives 4
treatment plan 36, 40
treatment room 160
treatment sessions 32–78
   age-appropriate 32
   blocks 33–4
   in groups 32–3
Twister 59

unilateral activities 141

ventricle shunts, children with 35
verbal contact 76
vestibular tolerance 49
vestibular-propioceptive processing 5
vestibular-proprioceptive activities 137–8
vestibular-proprioceptive stimulation 68
vision 104
vision screens 11
visual perception tests 23
visual space perception 142–3

Western Psychological Services 21
whingeing 83
withdrawal 84, 87
writing speed 25–6